STUTTERING
AND ITS
MANAGEMENT

WHAT THE BRAIN TELLS US

WILLIAM G. WEBSTER

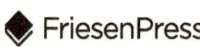 FriesenPress

One Printers Way
Altona, MB R0G 0B0
Canada

www.friesenpress.com

ISBN
978-1-03-831377-5 (Hardcover)
978-1-03-831376-8 (Paperback)
978-1-03-831378-2 (eBook)

1. HEALTH & FITNESS, HEARING & SPEECH

Distributed to the trade by The Ingram Book Company

TABLE OF CONTENTS

Dedicated with love and thanks to
Anne Godden-Webster,

my best friend, companion, advisor, and spouse,
who kept me on track and well-motivated by offering
to do the dishes and other chores so I could work
on the manuscript without interruption.

Speech is civilization itself. The word, even the most contradictory
[or disfluent*] word, preserves contact—it is silence which isolates.
Thomas Mann (1875-1955)
[**added by WGW*]

PREFACE

I am a person who stutters. I have always been a person who stutters, and I have come to accept that I shall always be a person who stutters. I am also a retired university professor and former dean. During my forty-nine years as a professor, I held academic and administration positions that required much talking and listening. There might seem to be a disconnect between these statements, but I hope this book will demonstrate that there really is not.

Two intersecting themes run through this book. The first theme is experiential, an account of my nearly 80-year **personal** relationship with stuttering and the unpredictable and seemingly chance encounters or events that shaped the path along which my **professional** relationship with stuttering evolved. The second theme, derived from that professional relationship, includes a discussion of my research on brain mechanisms underlying stuttering. The two key questions I explore in this second theme are: 1) What is different about the brain of the person who stutters? 2) What happens in the brain of the person who stutters that accounts for the marked variations in stuttering severity across time and situations? The book goes on to explore how the answers to these questions, together with the account of my personal experiences with stuttering, can inform strategies that people who stutter might adopt for the management of their speech.

The reader may legitimately ask if the research I will be discussing, much of it done a quarter century ago, is seriously out of date. Regrettably, I don't believe it is. Much of the more recent research on stuttering and the brain has used neuroimaging methodologies like positron emission tomography (PET) scans and functional magnetic resonance imaging (fMRI) technology to map regional brain activation associated with stuttering. Contrary to what was predicted by many in the early 1990s, research involving regional cerebral blood flow mapping has not yet shone as much useful light as hoped on the two key questions asked above. We know from those imaging studies that there are a number of areas of the brain that are "stuttering-related," areas that become activated or deactivated during stuttered speech. Unfortunately, the studies have told us little yet about how the different activated/deactivated areas actually contribute to stuttering and its management. I hope that readers will find the Two-Factor Interference Model outlined in the book to be as useful to them as I have found it for managing my own stuttering. The British statistician George Box wrote in 1976 that "All models are wrong, but some models are useful." The Two-Factor Interference Model, based on an experimental neuropsychology approach, is without doubt incomplete and hence wrong, but I would like to think it may still be useful for thinking about and responding to stuttering.

I have assumed that many readers of this book will have only limited familiarity with the nature of stuttering and its treatment, or with the study of brain mechanisms underlying behaviour in general and stuttering in particular, or with the nature of experimental neuropsychology. Accordingly, the two chapters on research include discussions of the rationale, assumptions, methods, and equipment used in the studies that are described. I want the reader to understand the link between the data and their interpretation, which requires some understanding of the method, because it is the method that gives the results. To facilitate such understanding, I have included in various places boxed "Reflection Notes" to encourage thinking about what the Model would say about questions and issues related to stuttering. I hope that readers will take the time to consider these questions and generate other questions themselves.

I have never been comfortable with describing people who stutter as "stutterers." I am more comfortable referring to myself and others who stutter as "people who stutter." For me, the former designation inappropriately defines us by our stuttered speech; the latter implies our stuttered speech is just one of many qualities or attributes we have as individuals. Throughout this book, I have tried to use "person who stutters" wherever possible. However, there are parts, particularly in chapters 5 and 6 on research, where the phrase "person who stutters" became too cumbersome for maintaining clarity and flow. Reluctantly I ended up resorting to "stutterer" in places. Similarly, although I respect and support an individual's choice of pronouns that best reflect their sense of self, I have generally used traditional pronouns so as to facilitate the flow of the prose in this book. Further on terminology, I have used the word "stutter" throughout the book despite there being another word, "stammer," that is used by some, particularly in the UK. I view the two words as synonymous.

Stuttering has impacted every aspect of my life. Sometimes the impact has been negative; at other times, I am pleased to report, stuttering had a positive impact or had positive consequences. As I look back over my life, I am most proud of having come to understand the nature of my stuttering and how to manage my speech. I have not found a cure for my stuttering, but I do manage stuttering reasonably well much of the time. That's almost as good.

My eldest daughter, Reiko Fuentes, first suggested that I write a book like this about my personal and professional journey. Her sentiments were strongly echoed by my other children, Yumi Webster, Heather Webster, and David Webster, who thought a book would help them and others get to know me and my work better. I hope this book will have broader appeal beyond family, including people who stutter together with their families and friends, neuroscientists, and speech-language pathology practitioners and students.

This book is also an acknowledgement of my gratitude to the people who were part of the many unpredicted and unpredictable, even seemingly random, twists and turns in my journey. Some of these people are identified but most are left anonymous. Without each of them, my journey would have been different and not as rich and fulsome. That journey has taken me from being a perplexed young person with little control over his speech to being a much older and hopefully wiser person who now manages his speech well enough much of the time. More importantly, I have found peace with the cards I was dealt. With gratitude, I acknowledge that, with the help of others, the cards turned out to have been a "full house." It is not my intention to offer much gratuitous advice to people who stutter, but I hope my story and the research findings that flow from it can encourage, inspire, or even empower.

I extend my special thanks to my good friend and Dalhousie University colleague, Dr. Joseph Byrne; to my retired speech-language pathologist friend in Montreal, Ms. Jill Harrison; and to my best friend, advisor, and spouse, Anne Godden-Webster, all of whom read and provided encouraging comments and observations on the manuscript at various stages of writing. Their assistance, together with that of the editors at Friesen Press, has been invaluable. In their reading, Joe brought the perspective of a clinical neuropsychologist and experienced book author, and Jill and Anne brought that of speech-language pathologists who have worked with children, adolescents, and adults who stutter. That said, any and all errors of fact or interpretation are mine alone.

William G. Webster, PhD

ABOUT THE AUTHOR

William G. Webster, PhD, is a retired university professor, a former dean, and a person who stutters. The first 22 years of his career included being a professor and chair of the Department of Psychology at Carleton University in Ottawa, Canada, where he established an active research program focused on brain mechanisms underlying stuttering. The results of that research have been published in journal articles and edited book chapters, have been presented at professional conferences, and form the core of this book. He co-authored with Marie Poulos in 1989 a clinical manual entitled *Facilitating Fluency: Transfer Strategies for Adult Stuttering Treatment Programs* (Tucson, AZ: Communication Skill Builders). In 1991, he was appointed Dean of the Faculty of Social Sciences at Brock University in St. Catharines, Ontario, and in 2002, Director of the School of Communication Sciences and Disorders at the University of Western Ontario (now Western University) in London, Ontario. From 2005 until his retirement in 2016, Will was Dean of the Faculty of Health Professions at Dalhousie University in Halifax, Nova Scotia. He has four grown children and resides in Halifax, Nova Scotia, with his wife, Anne.

INTRODUCTION

What Do We Mean by Stuttering?

This book is about stuttering, people who stutter, and the brains of people who stutter, and so the goal of this initial section is simply to describe briefly the nature of stuttering in a factual and objective way. In subsequent chapters, as I get into my life-long relationship with stuttering, I will discuss stuttering more from personal experiential and scientific perspectives. I will also share with you what I learned from my research about what is going on in the brain of the person who stutters and how that research can inform strategies for the management of speech by people who stutter. But, first, what do we mean by "stuttering?"

First, we think of involuntary disruptions to the flow of speech in children and adults. These include prolonged sounds at the beginning of syllables or words (e.g., prolongation of the m-sound in "mother"); blockages with little or no vocalization during the initiation of a word or phrase; repetitions of syllables or words or sounds (e.g., th-th-th-thanks); frequent use of a "starter" word or vocalization sound during the initiation of speech (e.g., uh-uh-thanks). Readers who have watched the film *The King's Speech* will have a good sense of the nature of these disruptions; they were well depicted. Sometimes the disruptions are so severe that it is difficult for the person who stutters to complete a sentence or for others to understand what is being said. More often, the speech does move forward but with lurches and disruptions. When stuttering is severe, communication is difficult for both the speaker and the listener.

These external characterizations of stuttering are what I and everyone else who stutters live with to one degree or another during our everyday lives. People differ in the frequency and severity of their stuttering, some having difficulty much of the time and others having difficulty only occasionally. Within the individual person who stutters, there is also variation of severity across time and situations. The severity can change from day to day, even moment to moment. It can also change with age. Dr. Charles Van Riper (1905-1994) was a well-known and influential speech pathologist who had a severe and persistent stutter and learned to control his speech well. He lamented that as he got into his senior years his stuttering became increasingly more frequent and severe.

People who stutter are affected in different ways by different situations. Situations that reportedly are **not** problematic for most people who stutter include talking when one is entirely alone, talking to a pet, or singing. Situations that commonly create difficulties include, for example, saying one's name; introducing others; using the telephone to ask for a specific person, or to say who is calling; speaking to people in authority; participating in Zoom meetings; ordering food at a drive-thru intercom; making a public presentation (although even some people who don't stutter report they would "rather die" than give a speech); or reciting or reading a passage in a public setting. People who stutter commonly can tell you not only which situations are particularly difficult for them, but which initial sounds are particularly difficult.

Sometimes stuttered speech is accompanied by facial tics or grimacing that reflect tension in the speech musculature when trying to force sounds or trying to speak without sufficient air in the lungs. These movements add to the tension and anxiety about speaking. They also add to how uncomfortable it can be for some people to listen to someone who is actively stuttering.

Associated movements can also occur verbally or with the hands or feet, and these are called "superstitious behaviours." This refers an utterance or behaviour that, at some time in the past, was followed immediately but coincidentally by a break in a block or by a period of sustained fluency. This leads the person, when stuttering, to repeat that utterance or behavior in the expectation that the same improvement in speech would recur, an expectation that is seldom realized except by chance or coincidence. For example, if during a stuttering block the person happened to utter a quick, "what-the," and this coincided with a release from the block, the person may continue to utter "what-the" when they next foresee difficult words or a block coming. Hence the characterization, "superstitious."

This body tension and these superstitious behaviours all amount to physical struggles in speaking that are acutely evident to the speaker and usually to the listener. This situation does not contribute to effective and satisfying communication. The experience of stuttering goes beyond the difficult words or sounds; it is influenced by the reactions of listeners to our stuttered speech. Reactions of others span the waterfront and can include, for example, signs of impatience; filling in a blocked word or a sentence; smirking; looking uncomfortable; or looking away or looking down. Fortunately, reactions are often ones of patience, understanding, and non-judgmental silence. Nothing is appreciated more by the person who stutters than these latter kinds of reactions.

The features of stuttering that I have just described are what one might call the **external** manifestations of stuttering. They occur in the public domain. They are objective, observable, and can be measured. But there is another whole dimension to stuttering: the **subjective experience of stuttering**, a domain that is private and much less evident to the conversation partner. But it is no less real.

In later chapters, I will suggest that much of the impact of stuttering on the life of the person who stutters comes from this **internal domain**. The nature of this domain was, for me, captured well by William H. Perkins who characterized stuttering as being, "the sense of an impending loss of control" (Perkins, 1983, 1985). In people who stutter, it is this sense that underlies the fears and anxieties that flow from or are caused by being blocked when speaking. The characterization captures the frustration of not being able to say what one wants to say, and the shame and humiliation of then being seen as incompetent, or even worse. And it is that sense of impending loss of control that leads to "holding back," the avoidance of situations or people or words or sounds that are problematic. If, when facing a speech situation, one has this sense, avoiding the situation entirely is one way (although ultimately not an effective way) to deal with the fear of a possible loss of control.

The person who stutters and who experiences this sense of impending loss of control is **not** in a constant state of fear and anxiety. They do not live in a constant state of free-floating anxiety. It is the **prospect** of speaking, or the **anticipation** of speaking, or the anticipation of possibly being called upon to speak, that triggers the sense of impending loss of control. The rest of the time this person is as free of fear and anxiety as anyone else. It is through the experience of a loss of voluntary speech control and the consequent fear and anxiety of it recurring, that stuttering has its ultimate impact on the person who stutters. One can be fluent at this moment but still fear a loss of control at the next. I should be clear at the outset that, although fear and anxiety may accompany stuttering, it is **not** fear and anxiety that caused stuttering in the first place. The wiring of the brain is the **initial cause** of stuttering; fear and anxiety are a **consequence**. That said, for reasons discussed in later chapters, fear and anxiety undoubtedly can and do add to the **severity** of stuttering.

These two domains, the external and the internal, the objective and the subjective, the overt and the covert, do not always covary systematically. In other words, usually a person who experiences a lot of blocks and struggle in their speech may feel, not unexpectedly, an intense sense of impending loss of control. But another person may not have that sense and just barges ahead, disfluencies and all. Still another a person who experiences only the occasional block and little struggle may still experience an intense sense of impending loss of control. With this latter person, even though the external speech disruptions may seldom occur, the fear that the disruptions might happen is still very real.

This internal experience of stuttering, referred to as **hidden or covert stuttering**, may often be dealt with through avoidance of one kind or another. In a "covert stutterer," external stuttering (i.e., speech disfluencies) may occur infrequently because the person is acutely tuned into upcoming speech challenges and circumvents them through avoiding particular words or sounds or situations. For example, rather than ordering what I really want, a "Big Mac" hamburger, I order "Chicken Nuggets" because the Ch-sound is easier for me to say than the problematic B-sound; or I go into the restaurant rather than use the more convenient drive-thru intercom, which is like the hated telephone. When I do these things, no one knows that I stutter, because my speech is not disfluent; I've avoided the problem words. As astonishing as it may be, occasionally even close friends and family members of someone who is a covert stutterer may be unaware that this person actually stutters. Anyone who thinks that people who stutter aren't smart or clever haven't thought about how difficult it can be cognitively and emotionally to not overtly stutter by using avoidance strategies alone. A speech-language pathology friend described a client of hers who, rather than phone, took a bus across town to come into the clinic to make an appointment for the next week. This kind of avoidance takes tremendous planning, time-management, and foresight.

Where does stuttering come from? Research dealing with the speech of identical twins who were reared apart indicate a clear genetically based predisposition to stutter. However, the findings also indicate that stuttering is not **determined** by genetics, only that it is **influenced** by genetics. The concordance of stuttering in such twin pairs (Howie, 1981; Kidd, 1984) is well below 100% (which is what it would be if the whole story were genetics) but substantially greater than the concordance for same-sex siblings. Experience (which could include intrauterine experiences or birth events) probably plays a role in some stuttering expression as I will comment on below. Maturation also plays a role. It is estimated that as many as 5% of preschool children will experience stuttering in some form, and about 80% of those children will grow out of it by six or seven years of age. This leaves an estimated 0.5% to 1% of the youth and adult population (4:1 ratio of males to females) as people who stutter. Chapter 6 includes a discussion of the important research by my former graduate student, David Forster, on the brain mechanisms associated with this maturation process.

There has long been speculation on possible differences in the etiology or origins of stuttering among stutterers who have a known family history of stuttering and those who do not. Poulos and Webster (1991) drew upon data from a clinical population of 189 adult and adolescent stutterers and found that 112 (66%) reported a **family history** of stuttering. Among these, only 3 (2.4%) reported any birth or early childhood factors or events that were thought by the person or their family to be associated with stuttering onset or that might have precipitated stuttering. Respondents were asked, among other things, specifically about any known prenatal difficulties, birth complications, accidents, or head injuries during early childhood. Twenty-one (37%) of the 57 respondents **without** a family history of stuttering reported such a factor or event.

The implication of these findings (and bearing in mind the many limitations that are associated with retrospective self-report studies) is that within a clinical population of adults presenting as people who have stuttered since childhood, there may be two etiologically different subgroups. One subgroup is thought to consist of individuals with a genetically inherited predisposition for stuttering. The second and smaller subgroup consists of individuals without a family history but who may have sustained some form of early brain trauma. I should add that a still smaller group would be comprised of adults who have sustained a head injury in adulthood and whose stuttering started at that time or shortly after. This is called **acquired stuttering** to contrast it from **developmental stuttering** which starts in childhood.

So, again, where does stuttering come from? Very briefly, it comes from the brain and, more specifically as I will discuss in chapters 5 and 6, it comes from how parts of the brain of people who stutter are interconnected. Except for a few exceptional cases of acquired stuttering, the brains of people who stutter are not damaged and, in a resting (non-speaking) state, show the same patterns of activation and deactivation found in their fluent peers. However, their speech motor control areas are vulnerable to interference from activity in other parts of the brain, and during speech this interference is manifest as stuttering and can be reflected in PET and fMRI brain scans. Understanding the origins and nature of the interference will suggest strategies that can be used to minimize interference and promote fluent speech.

PART I

The Early Years of a Boy/ Young Man Who Stuttered

CHAPTER 1

First Words and Early Days (1944-1961)

On Christmas Eve of 1946, thirteen days before my third birthday, I uttered my first word. I am told that I had quietly made my way to the decorated Christmas tree, took a wrapped package from under the tree, opened it, and declared "doggie." The dog in question was actually a small wooden pull-toy, a black dog with a red collar and red wheels. In light of the importance of speech sounds in my life, I still keep that toy dog on display at home, and greatly treasure it. I gather that my mother and father could not have been happier with that first utterance. Nearly three years of age was (and is) quite late to start speaking. They were beginning to suspect that my delayed speech was due to deafness; there was apparently no reliable way to test for deafness in infants at that time.

I do not know when my parents realized that speaking was a problem for me. It is also not clear whether my early speech production was more difficult for me or for them. My difficulties were not drawn to my attention. In fact, I cannot recall any time in my whole life when my parents had any discussion with me about stuttering. This may have reflected my father's discomfort with his own stuttering. More likely, though, it reflected the usual professional advice given at the time not to draw attention to the difficulties. Looking back, it seems to me that this approach turned what were speech production difficulties into *unmentionable* speech production difficulties. There must have been some not-so-subtle messages in that for me as a child.

Following the end of World War II, my family moved from Ottawa, where my father been stationed, to Montreal where my parents had lived before the war. My father had been an early professional psychologist in Canada (E.C. Webster et al., 2023), and right after the war he was re-establishing his private practice in vocational guidance and industrial psychology. He had also been appointed to the psychology department at McGill University to teach and supervise graduate students in industrial psychology. Through his new professional contacts, he learned of a speech therapist, Mrs. Mary Cardozo, who assessed and treated children who stuttered. Speech-language pathology, as the profession is now called, was in its infancy at the time. As I learned many years later, Mrs. Cardozo had started the Speech Therapy Clinic at the Montreal Children's Hospital in 1944 where she was director at the time of her retirement forty years later. By all accounts, Mrs. Cardozo was a colourful and dynamic leader, and she was behind the founding, in 1955, of the Société d'orthophonie et d'audiologie du Québec (Order of Speech-Language Pathologists and Audiologists of Quebec). She was also a leader in her profession nationally through her involvement with the Canadian Association of Speech-Language Pathologists and Audiologists (now called Speech-Language and Audiology Canada).

My older sister, Eleanor, remembers the family appointments with Mrs. Cardozo on Saturday mornings at the local Anglican church hall. Apparently, therapy included the use of flash cards with pictures and words on them. I recall also the use of doll play, presumably intended to prompt spontaneous speech. I have no memory of Mrs. Cardozo, although she must have had some impact on the family as I do remember her name being mentioned (mainly by my sister) on occasion over the years.

I have the sense that my therapy did not last long, possibly because I was not making sufficient improvement to warrant continuation. Like many of his generation who had lived through the depression and the war years, my father always worked long hours. My mother looked after the children; my younger sister, Marian, was newborn at the time. In light of this, it would not surprise me if time was viewed as too precious to allow for patience with stuttering treatment that was not showing results, but this is purely conjecture on my part. None of this was ever discussed with me. The only comment from my father about stuttering that I can recall is that "stuttering treatment does not work." I have no idea whether that comment related to his personal experiences or to mine.

Our home was in Montreal West, a middle-class English Protestant community on the Canadian Pacific Railway main line just west of Montreal proper. Several blocks from the house were my elementary school, Elizabeth Ballantyne School, and in the opposite direction across the railway tracks my high school, Montreal West High School. In elementary school we walked to and from school twice each day because everyone went home for lunch. I remember remarkably little about the first eight or ten years of my life (although writing this book has been helpful in reawakening some memories). Unfortunately, what few memories I have are in large part associated with negative experiences with stuttering. That said, I believe I was a happy and contented child as long as speech wasn't involved.

Like many others of my generation who stuttered, I was teased during my school years. Being somewhat overweight and not particularly athletic, as well as being a boy who stuttered, led to occasional hurtful taunts in the school yard and classroom or on the walk to or from school. Not being able to say my name easily when attendance was being taken or to answer the teachers' questions or to comment in class, I drew into a shell for a number of years and remember being prone to daydreaming. I recall having had only a small group of school yard playmates, no more than two or three regulars, and I was often off by myself. I usually walked to and from school alone, but I don't recall ever thinking that I was shunned or avoided by other kids in the class. I was happy to be alone with my thoughts or with just one or two other friends with whom I did not have to compete for airtime. I was not regularly bullied or the brunt of "jokes" about stuttering, but when those things did occur, they were hurtful. They are the incidents, as few as they may have been, that I remember to this day.

My recollection of elementary school is that the teachers were sympathetic and dealt with my stuttering as best they could, even if just by not calling upon me to speak in class. They were supportive in other circumspect ways as well. One instance that comes to mind was when, in Grade 5 or 6, the school was to put on a fantasy play that involved all the pupils in several classes. The play was called *Cigamsti*, "It's Magic" spelled backwards. Every part of the play except one involved speaking or singing. The one exception was the part of the King because, as the teacher explained to everyone when the roles were being assigned, the tradition in the Kingdom of Cigamsti was that the Queen ruled (as in the story, *Alice in Wonderland*) and made all the royal proclamations and did all the speaking for the Crown. The teacher went on to say that because of this tradition, the role of the King required someone with a special royal demeanor who could wave magisterially to the crowds as the royal carriage made its way through the streets of the kingdom. She said that after a lot of careful thought, she and her fellow teachers had decided that the pupil who had those special qualities and would be perfect for the role of King was me.

After weeks of rehearsal and preparation of sets, the play was performed to a large audience of students, siblings, and parents. It was a smash hit, as was the role of the King. I still remember the accolades from teachers and classmates' parents alike. Not a mention of stuttering, only magisterial demeanor and perfect waving, together with the impressive crown on my head. Having no speaking lines meant that during the rehearsals and the performance itself, I was free of that terrible sense of impending loss of control discussed in the Introduction. This was a wonderful experience in which I was comfortable in a performance context for the first time. I recognized that the adrenalin rush and the accolades at the end could become addictive.

As I look back, I am so grateful that the teachers handled this situation in such a sensitive and caring manner. I believe it made a real difference to how I was subsequently viewed by peers and parents alike, and it made a real difference in how I viewed situations with a spotlight on me. I realize now that, over the years, I benefitted in so many ways from being gently

18

pushed and supported by teachers and my mother to have a presence and to use my voice as best I could. But stuttering was **never discussed** or even explicitly mentioned.

According to report cards I still have, I did reasonably well academically. My lowest grade was for handwriting, and that grade was usually F (for Fair). I do remember once bringing home my report card with the usual F for handwriting, finding a dull blue pencil, and adding a stroke to turn the F into an E (for Excellent). I now understand the gentle glint in my mother's eyes when she reviewed the report card, but remarkably she said nothing. Nothing needed to be said. And it never recurred.

But school was a place where I lived in fear that I might be called upon and feel ashamed and humiliated by not being able to answer some simple question because of becoming blocked. By the time I reached Grade 7, I believe I was emerging from my shell, probably because I found the class material more interesting and because more of the work was done in writing with less reliance on oral participation in the classroom. But in some classes, there were still questions to be answered orally. I remember well, in Grade 6, actually raising my hand to answer a question posed by the teacher. Raising my hand was not something I often did, but in this case, I was sure of the answer. The teacher called my name, but I had been momentarily daydreaming with my hand raised and was surprised and startled when I heard my name. Once I realized what was happening, I got totally stuck on the initial sound in the answer. I still recall being briefly scolded for having raised my hand when I couldn't give the answer and then being passed over for another student. No wonder the sense of impending loss of control continued strong. Fortunately, there were not many instances like that which I can remember, but they hurt. And still no one talked to me about stuttering and how I felt about it. I was left to muddle through.

By the time I was in high school, my circle had increased somewhat, although I was never one of the cool kids and I never really had a close friend in whom I felt I could confide. The one constant "friend" I did have during all my school years was the family's English bulldog, Buster. He was the only living creature to which I could talk easily, and so, sitting on our back steps at home, I talked to him frequently, sharing my speech experiences and frustrations. I always felt Buster was quite empathic although probably skeptical of what I was saying about stuttering experiences because, since he was a pet, I had never actually stuttered when speaking to him alone.

In Grade 3, I had the opportunity to take violin lessons after school one day a week. I was intrigued by the violin, and my mother encouraged me. Understandably, progress was slow with school-based instruction, and my practicing was painful for all to hear. I am sure there were times when my mother rued the day that she had encouraged me to take lessons. Over the subsequent years, however, as I moved on to private lessons and my skills improved, playing the violin became a refuge from my stuttering. It allowed me to be on my own, in my room away from family and neighbourhood friends, and to not have to talk. After I had done the requisite practicing of scales and exercises each day, the violin provided a means for me to express my feelings—sometimes happy and cheerful, more often a little sad and lonely—with music that came from within, rather than from music books. As I moved the bow over the strings, generating the music as I went along, I felt a freedom that I never experienced with words. I sometimes tried to write the music down on paper, but seldom got beyond eight or ten bars. That was okay, because I remember thinking that it was not the recording of my music on paper that was important and satisfying, it was expressing my feelings to myself in the present.

My parents eventually bought me a really good violin and bow that set me on a path that required much greater commitment, both from me in terms of my practicing and from them in terms of the costs. My teacher for a number of years was Mr. Jan Charuk, a member of the Montreal Symphony Orchestra. He was a good teacher, but the challenge I had with him was that he wanted me to phone him the night before my Saturday lesson to confirm the time of the lesson. I dreaded Friday evenings because using the phone was so difficult. I could seldom ask to speak to Mr. Charuk by name when his wife answered, and when I finally got that out, I couldn't say my own name (even though it was clear to all who I was and why I was calling). At about this point in the "conversation," Mr. Charuk or his wife would finish my sentence and tell me the time I should come for the lesson. I now realize that they were trying to help me overcome my difficulties with the phone through practice, but it didn't help. It simply reinforced the idea that phones were to be avoided.

Over the years, from early school days through professional life, I often experienced people completing my words or sentences if I was stuck or even hesitated. I'm sure they intended to be helpful, but often I sensed simple impatience. The irony was that usually the word or phrase offered was not what I was trying to say, and so I would start over again and then get stuck in the same place. For those who were impatient, I could almost feel their eyes rolling. All quite amusing in retrospect but not at the time. The experience did nothing to contribute to feeling good about myself.

My music lessons with Mr. Charuk continued at what is now Le Conservatoire de Musique et d'Art Dramatique du Quebec in downtown Montreal. Most of the students were francophone, and it was an interesting time in Quebec's history when instruction and even informal conversations at the Conservatoire would often switch from French to English when an anglophone like me entered the room. I wanted to speak French, and I tried but without much success. My stuttering made my efforts to speak French quite futile. I also began to suspect that I was challenged with respect to processing the sounds of foreign languages, an idea I will return to in a later chapter.

I continued private lessons with Mr. Charuk at Le Conservatoire until the beginning of my second year at university, at which time I realized I had to choose between music and academics. At that point, I wasn't doing well with either. I chose academics, and I have no regrets. But I did not abandon the violin. I still play to this day, although I played more when my children were younger. Living in Nova Scotia, as I do now, my musical tastes have changed from classical to fiddle music. I'm enjoying the greater spontaneity and opportunities for improvisation that fiddle music provides and, especially at this stage of my life, the informal fun of it all.

My mother must have accepted the fact that I stuttered, was socially withdrawn, and did not speak much at home, including at the dinner table. I sensed, however, that she found painful how little I spoke with her at lunch or after school about my day. She was a former schoolteacher, and I now appreciate how much she would have enjoyed hearing about my day in school. In retrospect, I suspect that she encouraged me to do things like violin that would put me in a positive spotlight and that didn't involve speaking (reminiscent of *Cigamsti*). I was the only one in my class who had signed up for lessons in Grade 3, and I believe it gave me an identity other than, "the guy who stutters," among my friends, their parents, and the teachers at school. My mother was insightful, and seemed very pleased when friends or neighbours would comment approvingly on my music. My involvement with music today continues to contribute to an identity that goes far beyond my speech.

My mother also supported my joining the local hockey team for my age group. Because of my larger circumference, limited athletic abilities, and lack of proper hockey equipment, I was assigned to the high-profile position of goalie (for which the equipment was provided). The coach assumed that I would be able to readily block the net, and fast skating was not required. Also, since my skating skills were poor, it solved the potential problem for the coach of otherwise having to put me on the ice occasionally in a forward or defence position. I recall with amusement that, because of the heavy gear combined with my poor skating, my teammates had to pull me from one end of the rink to the other at the change of periods. As my mother hoped, the goalie position saw me stand out from the crowd, again contributing to an identity other than one based on speech. My mother and I laughed many years later about the fact that she paid a big price for encouraging me. Hockey in those days was played on outdoor ice surfaces, and so she had to stand in the snow in the cold Montreal winters (much colder than now) to watch me and cheer me on. Looking back on the time, I realize just what a supportive person my mother was for me in her own quiet way. She had her own challenges, being a post-war suburban housewife and, at least in her later years after her sister had died, suffering from loneliness and depression. I do wonder now if it would have been helpful, not only for me but also for her, if we had been able to have discussions about my stuttering and our respective feelings about it and its implications.

My hockey career ended at around age fourteen. My team was not winning often, due more to goals I let in rather than insufficient goals scored by our team. But mainly I was bored with hockey culture, in no small measure because I didn't feel comfortable trying to participate in fast-paced change-room banter. I just wanted to be away from boisterous and boasting peers and coaches.

Across the street from our home in Montreal West was a large United Church of Canada church with a formidable minister of Scottish heritage, Dr. G. Campbell Wadsworth. My mother was a person of faith who attended church regularly and who actively participated in a leadership capacity in various church functions. My father did not go to church at all. Interestingly, however, he and Dr. Wadsworth would often spend long periods of time talking on the sidewalk between the church and the house. I would love to have known what they talked about. The apparent incongruity always made me wonder if Dad was more spiritual than he appeared or acknowledged.

My mother took my two sisters and me to church and Sunday school every week. Going to church ultimately had a powerful impact on me, as I will discuss in chapter 3. I very much looked forward to church, because it gave me a chance to quietly pray for relief from my affliction. My prayers were not ones of gratitude; they were not for others; they were for me. I read parts of the Bible regularly looking for passages that might provide solace. However, I was not looking for solace; I was looking for an angel to visit me and cure me of my stuttering. I prayed long and hard in church every Sunday for many years. And I prayed most nights at home before going to sleep. My prayers were simple: stop the stuttering; let me say my name; let me use the phone; let me stand up in class and speak like the other kids. Nothing happened, including at Sunday School where I had hoped there might be some a temporary good behaviour reprieve granted for the day by an angel.

In my early teens, I thought one way to get God's attention and to be heard might be to demonstrate greater commitment by expressing the intention to become a minister in the church. However, I then realized there was no way I could give a sermon or read Bible passages or say prayers during a service without making the service interminably long, and so I didn't pursue that strategy. By the time I started university, my faith was diminishing as I slowly accepted that my prayers were not going to be answered. However, as I will return to in chapter 3, perhaps that angel did appear some years later after all. I just needed to be patient and open to what a "cure" might actually look like.

By the time I entered high school, I had thinned down physically and had developed more self-confidence. My speech seemed to have improved somewhat in informal social interactions, and I remember very few situations in which anyone made fun of my speech, except by my oldest and best friend at the time, Trevor Hughes. I always interpreted his put-downs to be simply a bizarre and psychopathic-type expression of friendship. But public speaking and asking questions in class continued to be highly problematic for me. I held back because of the constant sense of impending loss of control. Situations in which I had to introduce myself or use the telephone were equally problematic for the same reason.

The annual family Christmas party at the McGill University Faculty Club to which my father took the family was always a nightmare for me because of the greetings and introductions that were expected. It was a dreadful time as I could never say "Merry Christmas" as expected without getting hung up on the "M" sound of "Merry," or to say my first name without prolonging the "Wo" sound in "William" or repeating endlessly the "B" sound in "Bill." The Annual New Year's family party for Rotary Club members was not much better, although I did find the initial "Ha" sound of "Happy New Year" easier to say.

Christmas Day itself was never a favourite speech day. The low part of the day was making the customary long distance phone call from Montreal to my grandparents' home in Vancouver. There was only one phone in the house, so everyone had to speak sequentially to wish the grandparents a Merry Christmas and to thank them for the gift received. In those days, long distance phone calls were expensive, and so by the time I was put on the phone (usually, by implied mutual agreement, near the end of the call) there was considerable time pressure to speak quickly, which of course just magnified the difficulty of my stumbling over the required words. I never felt good after that call. The celebrations for the rest the day were with aunts, uncles, cousins, parents, and siblings. It was good to feel part of an extended family, but I remember few other things about Christmas days because my strategy for dealing with them was to withdraw to the extent I could.

Notwithstanding these disheartening social occasions, I continued to find myself encouraged or pushed into situations with spotlights that contributed further to my being seen as more than "the kid who stutters." In Grade 10, I was asked by the vice-principal of the school if I would be a member of the student council. After I agreed to do so, I was asked to be the vice-chair. At least it didn't seem as if this position would require much speaking, because the meetings were led by the chair, and a teacher guided the discussions.

One of the council projects for the year was to update its constitution, but the new constitution needed to be presented to the student body for adoption. The school principal felt that this presentation should be led by the vice-chair of the council, since the chair had been so involved with making the revisions. Interestingly, I did not back away from this "suggestion" and agreed to do the presentation. By that time, I was realizing that, although *ad lib* talking or speaking off-the-cuff continued to be very difficult and was to be avoided, my speech could be somewhat fluent if I was lucky on the day and was well prepared. Good preparation allowed me to know exactly what I needed to say word-for-word and to focus more on how to say the words rather than what words I should say. I had been learning that slower and well-articulated speech, if I could just remember to do it, was helpful for facilitating fluency.

As it turned out, somehow there was virtually no stuttering in my speech during that presentation to the large auditorium of students and teachers about the proposed constitution! And there were even a couple of questions to field from the audience. I still remember clearly standing on the stage and reading slowly into the microphone and having what could only be described as an "out-of-body experience." I seemed to be observing myself and wondering who the person on the stage really was. Surely it wasn't me, "the guy who couldn't say his name." As it ended, I felt elated and almost stunned by the clapping and the wonderful experience of success. It was the first time I had had that experience (although *Cigamsti* in elementary school was an approximation, but that had not required any speaking on my part), and I'm pleased to say it was not the last. In the years that followed, I had a few other similarly liberating and energizing experiences, but that one, the constitution presentation, sticks in my memory for having shown me what might be possible. And it was my introduction to the idea of not avoiding a situation out of fear of stuttering. It would be many years, however, before I could fully accept and implement that non-avoidance strategy.

After the presentation, many of my fellow students congratulated me and commented on how fluent I had been, and several teachers did so as well. It was a wonderful turnaround from the teasing or stuttering imitations or other put-downs that were the more usual (even if infrequent) reactions to my speaking. It was also a particularly wonderful turnaround from the self-criticism and self-blaming that usually followed my speaking in public. One of the teachers went on to suggest that I should consider joining the debating club in the school. At first, I thought she was making a joke, but in fact she was serious. I was flabbergasted but intrigued. So, I took her suggestion to visit the debating club which was about to meet that afternoon. When I arrived at the room, the club had just got underway. The teacher running the club, who had not been at the constitution presentation, chastised me for being late and wanted to know what I wanted. When I tried to explain, all I could do was block on the initial words. In a dismissive, almost disgusted tone, the teacher told me just to sit down and be quiet. The debating club was not for me; the elation of success was gone and much of the appeal of avoidance was resurrected.

As I reflect on how I was encouraged and pushed by my mother and by teachers, I realize how beneficial this was both for my self-esteem and for having to do the one thing I feared more than any other—speaking. I began to realize by then that my speech was often better than what I feared it might be. And when I was forced to speak, I sometimes learned things I might try to do (or not do) to improve my speech or presentation in the future.

My circle of friends slowly expanded, and this occasionally included a girl. I remember in Grade 9, after consulting with my older sister about what one actually talks about with a girl, I tried phoning a girl in another class to ask if I could take her to one of the regular Friday evening dances at the school or local church hall. I hung up the phone immediately when I couldn't even get out an initial sound to ask to speak with her. This was not an unusual experience for me with the phone. I felt badly and went to the dance alone. I think I did ask a girl there for a dance, and we might have exchanged a few words. Although I went to a good number of school dances over those years, I don't recall any other attempts at a date until high school graduation.

In the fall of Grade 11, the final year of high school in Quebec, the graduation ceremonies and dinner dance were still on the distant horizon, but I thought I should decide soon who to invite as it might take me a while to get up the courage to try this kind of phone call again. I didn't want to risk everything on a phone call and so, when an opportunity presented itself for me to approach in the school hallway the particular girl I had in mind, I did so, and I invited her to be my date the following June. Much to my surprise, she accepted my invitation on the spot, although I suspect it was because she was so stunned by an invitation to a dinner-dance that was more than six months away. I say this because, a few weeks later, when I invited her to a movie, she turned me down. I interpreted this as reflecting some regret on her part at having committed herself so early in the year. But regardless, I recall we both had a good time at the dinner dance, although neither of us said very much. She was quiet herself, but she had a lovely smile.

What made it all a little awkward was that sometime in the spring of 1961, just before graduation, I met a girl from a different school at a house party. She had a wonderful and engaging speaking style which seemed to make my speech come more easily. And I rather liked her. As importantly, she had a name that started with a sound I could usually say without blocking. I had an opportunity to tell her I would phone (so she would be forewarned), and my first attempt at a phone call was reasonably successful. We had a first date, to a local school dance. Another highlight of elation! However, it was a little awkward to explain why I wasn't asking her to the graduation dinner dance to be held by the school a few weeks later. However, she and I continued to go out together for some time after that. As it turned out, many years later and under circumstances I will return to in chapter 8, she played a pivotal role in shaping the directions of my professional career. Yet another one of those unforeseeable and unpredictable circumstances that shape a life.

In Grade 11, I was asked to be the editor of the yearbook that year. Again, I now see that this was an activity that set me apart from the other students and made me something more than "just the kid who stutters." I also suspect that the offer was influenced by teachers quietly supporting me because of my speech difficulties. Being yearbook editor was a great experience requiring talking regularly with the various assistant editors, and that contributed to my growing profile, self-confidence, and self-esteem. And for reasons I didn't understand, that seemed to help my speech. Speaking extemporaneously was still very difficult, but by this time many one-on-one and small group conversations were becoming more manageable, at least on "good days." I was able to arrange things so I didn't have to use the phone much—that was the domain of the assistant editors to whom I delegated those responsibilities. Avoidance was still my good friend.

I have often reflected on the contrast between my difficulties with extemporaneous talking and the apparent ease with which others seem to do it. I now understand that I had been so focused over the years on the **how** of speaking or on the **avoidance** of speaking that I didn't focus sufficiently on the what. To speak extemporaneously requires having thought about, either beforehand or quickly at the time, what one might want to say about the topic at hand. It is difficult to do that if one is consumed with thinking mainly about the initial sounds of words that might be problematic. Only much later in life did I intentionally sit down to begin to figure out what my position might be on the issues of the day or at work. I also learned later in life that, contrary to my earlier belief, I was **not** in fact an active listener who paid attention well to what was being said. Just because I wasn't speaking at the moment did not mean I was listening. Instead, I was thinking about that sense of impending loss of control when I might need to say something in response. In a sense, I wasn't really part of a conversation. So, I learned that not only did I need to have my own thoughts on issues, I needed to be attending to what my conversation partner was saying and how that fit with my own views about the matter being discussed. It took me a long time to realize that the same principle applied to asking questions and learning from others. Again, being consumed with the **how** of speaking can be incompatible with the **what**. If I don't know

28

what I want to say or what I want to ask, the **how** of saying it becomes somewhat beside the point.

The final provincial examinations for Grade 11 included an oral exam in French. It was administered by our classroom teacher whom I remember as a kind and gentle woman and who, I believe, had a good understanding of what my verbal world was like. During the exam, she asked the questions slowly in French (of course) but there were several questions for which I honestly did not know the words I needed for the answer or, for that matter, what a good answer might actually be. All I could do at that point was to voluntarily switch into pretended spasms of blockages and repetitions embellished with facial twitches. This all prompted my teacher, in her kindness, to fill in words for me so I could finish an answer. Even now, more than sixty years later, I feel somewhat sheepish and guilty about having done that but, as my kids used to say, what else could I do? I passed the exam, and I retain fond memories of this kind teacher and of her efforts. Many years later, while on sabbatical leave from Carleton University, my continuing positive attitude towards spoken French, together with my realization that if I was going to live and work in Ottawa I needed to be able to speak French, led me to try to develop some oral French proficiency. This is described more fully in chapter 8. Although my written French and reading were passable, I eventually gave up trying to speak the language as I found I simply couldn't process the sounds. I have resigned myself to being a unilingual Canadian, and I hope that this is not just another one of my avoidance tactics.

* * * * * * * *

During this period of my life and during the following four years at McGill, summers were spent at summer camps.

My time at YMCA Kamp Kanawana, in the Laurentians north of Montreal, started with two-week stays beginning when I was seven years old. By the time I was in high school the stays were four or eight weeks long depending on whether there was to be a family beach vacation in Maine. Camp was a wonderful experience in terms of having to navigate new people and situations despite my feeling very much alone at times. This was not an entirely unwelcome feeling because being alone meant not having to speak. In contrast to school, few at camp seemed to care about my stuttering, perhaps because speaking was seldom required. I was just seen as being "a quiet and nice kid," not one who couldn't say his name without blocking.

The summer before high school graduation was spent on staff at Camp Nominingue, a private boy's camp also in the Laurentians north of Montreal. That was my first year at that camp. My father had been a Rotary Club friend of the camp owner and director, Mr. F.M. Van Wagner, and it was suggested to my father that I should send Mr. Van Wagner my resume. I did so and this was followed by a positive interview (I recall that Mr. Van Wagner did most of the talking), and I was hired as a counsellor-in-training who could contribute to the campcraft and canoe trip programs. I was ready for a change from the YMCA camp. I felt I needed new people (campers and staff), new routines, and opportunities to learn new ways of doing things. I worked at Camp Nominingue for a memorable five summers while I completed my final year of high school and then my undergraduate degree at McGill.

In the first summer at Camp Nominingue, I took the step of changing the name I called myself from "Bill" to "Will." It was (is) far easier for me to say. Although "William" and "Will" have the same initial sound, I have always found saying "William" to be more difficult than "Will," perhaps because "William" is multi-syllabic and presents more of a challenge to the left hemisphere speech motor control mechanisms as I will be discussing in chapter 5. Anticipating that discussion and moving momentarily to the right hemisphere, my difficulty with saying "William" may also have reflected the interfering effects on speech of many years of negative experience trying to say that name.

As I look back on those summers, I cared less about stuttering than I had at home. I simply barged ahead when I was talking with my tent group or giving instruction on campcraft (which had a lot of demonstrating rather than just talking), and I don't recall difficult and humiliating speech disasters. I smiled a lot, was cooperative and compliant, and generally didn't speak except when I had to. And I still had that sense of impending loss of control when things got a little more structured or formal. Perhaps what changed was I did not have the same fear of potential negative consequences and less motivation to avoid or withdraw from situations that involved speech. When I worked at Camp Nominingue, the one difficult speech day for me each summer was when I was assigned to have "Officer of the Day" duties. These duties included waking up the camp in the morning, ringing bells for activities during the day, watching for and greeting any visitors arriving at the camp, and, most challenging by far, saying Grace in the dining hall for the whole camp for each of the three meals. Based on how long it took me to begin to say each Grace to thank God for his bounty, the campers must have wondered if there actually was going to be any bounty for that meal or if I was protecting the chef who may have burned the porridge or the carrots or something equally dire. I did get through it.

Camp was generally a carefree time. I found the outdoors spiritually calming and uplifting, and being in the outdoors really did allow me to forget about stuttering. I loved the silence of nature. At that time, I could imagine myself being a forest ranger in the wilderness watching for smoke from my tower—although I realized that using the radio to report smoke or fire could be problematic with disastrous consequences. So much for that vocational option. I became skilled at using a canoe, and eventually I was co-leading wilderness canoe camping trips in La Verendrye Park. I discovered I was a good counsellor, a good teacher of campcraft skills, and could lead canoe trips well. I found speaking individually to my tent group was easier than in many contexts, possibly because I was more comfortable talking to people younger than myself rather than to authority figures. This experience provided a glimmer of hopeful light coming into the tunnel of life that lay ahead.

I began to view myself more positively as a skilled, competent, and accomplished person, a sense that was reinforced by others. This made stuttering somewhat less central to my self-image and projected identity, just as playing the violin had. Both camps included weekly Sunday morning chapel in their activities, and these provided me with fresh opportunities to pray for relief from my affliction, even though at camp the affliction was not one of "biblical proportions" as it often seemed to be at home. Camp really was something of a refuge. Unfortunately, as the summer days got shorter, there was the inevitable return to the city and to school.

* * * * * * * *

By the end of high school, I had learned a number of things about my stuttering, and few of them were good. I had come to believe that my stuttering was likely to continue; I would never be able to speak on the phone intelligibly; vocations that involved public speaking or making use of telephones or radios were essentially closed to me; avoidance and procrastination were useful short-term strategies (but, as I later learned, terrible long-term ones); and no angel was going to come to cure my speech. I didn't know what I would do with my life when I couldn't even reliably say my name. But while I believed all that to be true, I wouldn't accept it. I just wanted to get on with things without dwelling on my speech. I tried with some success to think about stuttering only when I was speaking or anticipating doing so. I generally didn't think much about stuttering when I was alone.

At this time, I felt increasing anger at the world and at myself, and that would burst forth on occasion in unfortunate and selfish ways. For example, I had somehow found that if I intentionally created a fuss in a restaurant or store, speaking loudly and forcefully and acting outraged about poor service or poor food, my speech became almost stutter-free. That result was sufficiently energizing for me to seek out opportunities to be, frankly, a verbal bully. I now look back on this phase, which fortunately did not last long, with considerable shame. The people on whom I took out my anger and bad feelings about myself had not teased me or reacted to my stuttered speech or done anything disrespectful, and I had no business treating them the way I did. I owe them an apology. Despite the quiet support I felt at home from my mother and at school from most teachers, I did not like myself. It is no wonder that within a few years I found myself drawn to alcohol, a deliberate (and unsuccessful) effort to reduce my stuttering, reduce the pain and anger associated with it, and assuage the guilt I had about my occasional lashing out at those around me.

It not a good place to be as I finished high school and started my undergraduate years at McGill.

CHAPTER 2

Laying the Foundation:
Undergraduate Years (1961-1965)

McGill University was always in the family blood. Both of my parents were McGill alumni, my father held a professorial appointment at the university, and my sister, Eleanor, was part of the first graduating class of McGill's Bachelor of Science of Nursing program. It was always assumed that if I were to attend university it would be at McGill. And yet, during my first year there, I felt lonely and isolated.

I knew few people in my classes and continued to avoid social occasions. I decided not to join a fraternity, mainly because I found it so difficult to participate in the loud and hurried banter during the annual fraternity recruitment week. I continued to live at home that year and I was driven to the campus each day by my father, although we spoke little since he used the travel time to plan his day. My classes were large, although some had smaller seminar groups in which, of course, I spoke little. Most of my interactions that year were with students I had known in high school. Although I liked them and could speak fairly easily with them, they were still part of my old life. At this time, just prior to the Cuban missile crisis in 1962, many of my classmates and I were anxious by what seemed to be the very real prospect of nuclear war. I was drawn to writing poetry, was drifting and not terribly engaged in my classes, and was not doing well academically. I remember my mother expressing concern that I might lose the "faculty bursary" award that covered most of my tuition. Continuation of the bursary required maintaining a good academic average. Mine had become borderline, but good enough to keep the bursary the following years. It was not a great start to university days.

With one key change, my second year was the beginning of a new phase of my university life with more hope. The university had just opened new residence halls for male students, and my parents thought it would be good if I were to live in residence rather than at home. My decision at the time to major in psychology may have contributed to that decision. My father was Chair of the Department of Psychology, and he was concerned that if I continued to live at home any dinner table talk about his colleagues, who were my professors, could be problematic. Regardless of the motivation, being in Gardner Hall was one of the best things that could have happened to me. It forced me to be on my own, to look after myself, to speak for myself the best I could, and to interact with people in the dining hall and the residence building itself. I found that informal speaking around the residence was somewhat easier than informal speaking had been in earlier years. Looking back, I think my speech was improving but mainly in that residence context. No one seemed to care much that I stuttered. They seemed more interested in what I might have to say than in how I was saying it; unfortunately, I don't recall being good at providing much interesting commentary. Much of the speech pressure now came from within me (that sense of impending loss of control) rather than from others. I still look back with amazement that for most of my third year I worked on the telephone switchboard in the residence hall on Sunday evenings, answering the phone and taking messages. What seems to have made a difference for me was that the required social scripts were sufficiently few, simple, predictable, and repetitive that I was able to be reasonably fluent much of the time. Also, Sunday evenings were generally not a busy time for the switchboard.

Majoring in psychology in this second year also proved to be a great choice. Attending classes was an exciting and energizing experience for me. The psychology courses opened my eyes to new ideas about brain organization, consciousness, perception, and cognition, and I was fascinated by what I was learning. However, despite all the focus on brain-behaviour relations, it took another fifteen years before it dawned on me that stuttering might have an anomalous brain organization underlying it. My course in comparative anatomy prepared me to understand principles of evolution and the relationships among different vertebrate species, and this laid part of the groundwork for what I would work on ultimately for my doctoral studies. And my philosophy course in ethics prepared me to have the courage to abandon, out of ethical concerns, the research directions I would eventually start in the future that used laboratory animals as research subjects.

In all these courses I remained quiet and shy and did not ask questions or participate in the small group in-class discussions. It was a different feel than in the residence environment. Nevertheless, friends and instructors seemed to like me, perhaps due to my smiling and positive disposition, and that carried me far. Unlike in high school, questions were not directed by the instructors to individual students but were asked of the whole class. It was up to each student to raise their hand and often to be assertive. I seldom did so. Although I found my years at McGill really stimulating, I know I missed out on many opportunities to really explore and understand matters because of this reticence to ask questions and express opinions. Again, I was so consumed with **how** I might ask a question that I spent no time thinking about **what** I would ask and what I might contribute to the class discussion. And by the time I knew what and how I might make a comment or ask a question, it was too late because the topic of conversation had changed. To this day, even when my speech is good, I am still reticent to ask questions because of that pervasive sense of impending loss of control.

At this time, I was also beginning to realize something about the power of writing. Although I had difficulty expressing myself orally, writing was a different story, and increasingly, for good and bad, I started to take advantage of that. The good part was that I found a means to express myself, and

I could be eloquent and forceful; the bad part was that writing replaced trying to speak. It became another means of avoidance. I had not yet appreciated that writing and speaking are in fact two very different means of communication that can convey very different things above and beyond the words. I'll have more to say on this in chapter 8.

* * * * * * * *

The course that had the most immediate impact on my choices around the future was one which required completion of a research project. I did my project under the supervision of Mr. Cecil Baber, the manager of Advertising and Marketing Research at DuPont of Canada, located in downtown Montreal. Sometime earlier, Cecil had contacted the chair of the psychology department, who happened to be my father, to explore possibilities for a psychology undergraduate student to do some research with the company's advertising group. Cecil was committed to the idea that academic research should find application in the real world, that students are bright and have a lot to offer organizations like his, and that students would benefit from experiencing how theoretical concepts can actually be applied. He would have been a strong proponent of what we now call co-op education or experiential learning.

DuPont is a major global corporation and, in the 1960s, the head office of its Canadian operations was located in Montreal. Its main product lines at the time included cellulose films and textile fibres, including nylon. My impression was that most of the actual consumer advertising and market-ing activities were done in support of the Montreal fashion industry that used DuPont's fibre products.

Being a professional psychologist as well as an academic, my father shared Cecil's views about university-industry relations, and he committed to try to find a student on a trial basis. Dad approached me about doing my research project with Cecil at DuPont. I liked the idea and so I con-tacted Cecil's office by phone and arranged to meet with him in person (my preferred mode of interaction). The research project he proposed involved a comparison of the recall of information that had been presented visually vs. auditorily. This was seen as an important question at the time because television advertising was still relatively new compared to radio or newspaper advertising. The project went well—although the results were not particularly groundbreaking—and I was offered a job for the summer at DuPont in its advertising and marketing research group. This proved to be life-changing through being **speech-changing**.

I was to spend each of the eight weeks teaching myself about a different aspect of the social psychology research being carried out at the time by Dr. Carl I. Hovland (1912-1991) at Yale University. The focus was on attitudes, attitude change, and persuasive communications, all relevant to advertising and marketing and part of mainstream social psychology at the time. Then, at noon on the Friday of the week, I was to become a teacher and give a one-hour presentation on what I had learned that week about one aspect or another of Hovland's research and its potential implications for advertising and marketing. The audience usually included six or eight people drawn from DuPont, and another three or four who were friends of Cecil's from other firms in downtown Montreal, like Canadian National Railways and CIL. This presentation was then followed by a discussion among the group members (the "students") focusing on the implications of the research for their respective advertising and marketing efforts. Members of the group were all outgoing, loved talking, and liked one another which meant I did not need to do much speaking at that point in the proceedings. I was delighted to yield the floor and to listen to the interesting and animated discussions!

These eight weeks were a transformational experience in that they forced me to speak publicly on a regular basis, and they taught me that I could do a credible job of a presentation if I were thoroughly prepared. I recognized the importance of having confidence in what I was talking about and of organizing the presentation so it flowed smoothly with good transitions. I also learned the importance for me of using flipcharts or other means of visual presentation that I could fall back on to write a word if I got hung-up on saying it. The flip charts, largely prepared ahead of time, included the organization of the talk and key words to which I could point or circle or underline if needed. Somehow, I had the impression that people who give talks in public do so extemporaneously; being disabused of that idea was empowering. Such people are just well-prepared and have thought about **what** they want to say. I was spending far too much time worrying about **how** I was going to say it, but I needed to.

The following summer, right after I had graduated from McGill, I again worked for DuPont, but this time I was involved in consumer-related marketing research projects, most of which were survey and interview based. I was not involved with doing interviews myself, but my work still involved presentations of results to groups. Cecil was a wonderful mentor for me, and I suspect he hoped that I would go into advertising research as a career. He encouraged this by sending me for a couple of days to the DuPont head office in Wilmington, Delaware, to meet his counterparts. I don't think I impressed them because I could not keep up with the verbal banter of that team. Nevertheless, those two brief summers at DuPont were decisive for my future directions.

My interest in what I had been learning about attitude formation and change and persuasive communications, together with the positive response I had from Cecil and his colleagues to my lunch hour presentations, led to my decision to apply to graduate school to study social psychology. My initial thought had been to prepare to work in an advertising and marketing research capacity, but I soon began to harbour thoughts that I might be able to actually become an academic and be engaged in research and even classroom **teaching**! The brother of a colleague of my father was a professor of social psychology at Cornell University and he had a good reputation, and Dad suggested he might be a good person for me to work with. So, I prepared an application for admission to Cornell for graduate studies.

During my time at DuPont, I had also come to modify my stuttering in some situations by "bouncing" across hesitations and blocks, still being disfluent but keeping the sound stream moving. I wasn't doing bouncing intentionally, and indeed I was not even aware of doing this until nearly fifteen years later when, after a presentation at a conference on stuttering, several speech-language pathologists in the audience congratulated me on my skilled use of the bounce technique. The technique worked best when I was not aware of doing it and the bouncing occurred spontaneously, but over time I did learn how I could do this voluntary stuttering (bouncing) reasonably well. I also found that while it helped during public presentations, it did not work well with phone calls or with introductions. But it was another "arrow in my quiver" to help me get through some speaking situations.

During my final year at McGill, I was nominated for a Woodrow Wilson Fellowship established by the Woodrow Wilson Foundation (recently renamed the Institute for Citizens & Scholars) in the United States. The fellowships were intended to support first year graduate students in Canada and the United States planning to go into university teaching. I must confess that in proceeding to the interview in Boston, I felt like a fraud or an imposter. I wasn't convinced I could actually teach at the university level. I surmised that university teaching must be different from teaching a few marketing managers at DuPont during their lunch hour or early-teen boys at a summer camp. However, perhaps I was using the bouncing technique well in the interview, because the interview committee clearly didn't see any impediment; I was offered one of the 1000 scholarships awarded across North America. It would cover my tuition and living expenses. I was later offered admission at Cornell, including an enhanced award in recognition of my Woodrow Wilson Fellowship. It was an offer I couldn't refuse.

CHAPTER 3

Preparing for Neuroscience Research: Graduate Studies (1965-1970)

I n August 1965, I left Montreal in my newly acquired 1960 Volkswagen bug (thanks to my summer job with DuPont) and arrived at the main Cornell campus in Ithaca, New York. I immediately felt welcomed. I didn't really understand it at the time, but evidently there was prestige for universities to have Woodrow Wilson Fellows in their graduate programs. As well, the award freed the university from having to offer me, as a graduate student, the usual teaching or research assistantship, and it freed me from having to work twenty hours per week. Although the Woodrow Wilson Fellowship only covered the first year, the dean of graduate studies informed me that the university would guarantee me funding as a teaching assistant for my second and third years and then would award me the equivalent of another Woodrow Wilson Fellowship with no work responsibilities for my final year of studies. I did not appreciate then as I do now just what an unusual and wonderful opportunity this fellowship provided. I was also offered the opportunity to move directly into the doctoral program in social psychology before completing my master's work.

My future was unfolding in ways I could never have imagined when I was working those summers at DuPont.

I was also welcomed because of the hope by some at Cornell that, as a Canadian student, I might join its intercollegiate hockey team! Most of the Cornell team was made up of Canadian students, and there apparently had been some chatter about the fact that I had once played the goaltender position, and in Montreal (at that time the hocky capital of the world) to boot. However, I was at Cornell for a different purpose.

I lived in Sage Hall, a graduate residence with a cafeteria intended for graduate students, and I actually began to make friends fairly readily at mealtime. These were really bright students from a variety of disciplines, some of which I had never even heard of before. Almost everyone was new and was anxious to get to know others, and most of them loved to talk. And they were interesting. I could feel my horizons expand. But despite my real interest in the conversation, for all the usual reasons I was still quiet, held back, and asked few questions. As I look back on that year, I do think my speech was gradually improving in many situations, but I still feel badly about how little I contributed to most of those cafeteria conversations. As was the case when I lived in Gardner Hall, I was still haunted by that sense of impending loss of control which kept holding me back. I felt that if I were to overtly stutter at the cafeteria table, I might be exposed as the fraud I still thought I might actually be. My fears were not realized, and I made a few good friends in diverse disciplines and seemed to be able to speak with them easily. Another positive sign for the future.

Within a few days of arriving in Ithaca, I was to meet with my professor. It was only then I learned that he was on sabbatical leave and away from the campus for the year. Another professor had agreed to supervise me. I realized right away, however, that I would be doing my research for the next four years under the supervision of this new professor rather than the one originally planned. That, in turn, would lock me into a research stream that did not much interest me. Frankly I did not like the new professor, and I sensed he did not take a liking to me, perhaps because I didn't appreciate his research program (probably because I did not understand it at the time). After all that I had learned about attitude change and behaviour while at DuPont, his particular area of study in social psychology seemed dry, picayune, and very "academic" and did not inspire me. My initial enthusiasm about being at Cornell was starting to wither.

Within another week, classes began. At least eight other social psychology students, some new and others continuing, were enrolled in the fall term social psychology graduate seminar. Our classes were augmented by a few graduate students in sociology. As someone who stutters, I was impressed and intimidated by how much graduate students in social psychology and sociology talked. As a Canadian, I was equally impressed and intimidated by how assertive and self-confident the American students were. I could seldom get the floor to talk, and when I did, I was cut off almost immediately at my first hesitation. I must have been seen as a shy and withdrawn student who had nothing interesting to say rather than as a person who stuttered. Some weeks later, a fellow student (with whom I had become a "sort-of" friend) commented to me bluntly that I had an impressive pedigree but there was a mismatch with reality (ouch!). Within a week of that first class, it became apparent to me that I could never be a social psychologist, because I could never talk fast enough or fluently enough. So, my initial enthusiasm about being at Cornell was not only withering but starting to fall off the vine.

By pure chance I stumbled across, in the student lounge, a book called *Interhemispheric Relations and Cerebral Dominance* edited by Vernon B. Mountcastle, a well-known neurosurgeon and researcher from Johns Hopkins University. The book was a compilation of presentations made at a conference held in 1962 on current research dealing with differences in structure and function between the two cerebral hemispheres of the human brain. I was absolutely captivated. I literally couldn't put the book down and found myself repeatedly re-reading chapters so I wouldn't miss anything. Also, I felt proud that the conference had had such a strong Canadian representation among the contributors.

Different chapters focused on different research methodologies. These included the study of the effects of left and right hemisphere brain damage on perception, memory, and consciousness; assessing cerebral dominance using the Wada technique developed at the Montreal Neurological Institute by Dr. Juhn Wada; the analysis of processing of information (visual, auditory, tactual) directed primarily to one hemisphere or the other in neurologically intact people; and research on "split-brain patients." I will return to discuss some of these methods in later chapters.

I was particularly captivated by the studies of patients with intractable epilepsy who had had the corpus callosum sectioned in the midline to restrict epileptic seizures to one hemisphere (Sperry, 1974). By way of background, the sensory and motor systems are connected to the two hemispheres of the brain in such a way that it is possible to restrict some sensory information and some motor control to one hemisphere or the other. Since cutting the corpus callosum has the effect of disconnecting the hemispheres (the cerebral cortex) from one another, the cognitive processing capability of each hemisphere working alone can be assessed. When this is done, the complementarity of hemisphere specialization becomes readily and dramatically apparent within individuals. In general terms, tasks involving speech and language are far better performed when the sensory input is directed to the left hemisphere rather than the right. In contrast, tasks that involved visuo-constructional skills, such as arranging blocks in certain spatial configurations, are performed far better when the person is using the left hand (controlled by the right hemisphere) rather than the right hand (controlled by the left hemisphere).

According to the dogma of the time, non-human species were assumed to have symmetric brains, in other words, no unique specialized cognitive functions in one hemisphere vs. the other as found in the human brain. Given what I knew about evolutionary processes, I thought it implausible for human and non-human brains to be so fundamentally different. It seemed to me that this dogma was simply an updated version of efforts to differentiate the human species from all others, previous versions having been predicated on, for example, the possession of a soul or of a rational mind. This skepticism would impact my research in the near future.

At the time, I did not recognize how this chance encounter with the Mountcastle book and the ideas in it would so completely shape my future research and teaching career, and ultimately my understanding of stuttering. I quickly realized that I wanted to learn more about the functions of the cerebral cortex and how it processed information. But I also quickly realized that to go down that path was to forget about social psychology and attitude change and focus instead on my newly acquired interest in neuroscience. This interest had a strong foundation laid in me through several of my undergraduate psychology courses at McGill taught by Dr. Donald Hebb, Dr. Ronald Melzack, and Dr. Peter Milner, all eminent neuroscientists, and through the reputation of McGill and the associated Montreal Neurological Institute (MNI) both of which were on the forefront of the neurosciences.

When I returned to Montreal during the Christmas break in December, I was fortunate to meet with Dr. Hebb who advised me on universities at which there were active research programs related to cortical function. He also advised me to complete a master's thesis at Cornell as soon as possible and then move to another university for doctoral studies in physiological psychology. From his perspective, the subject matter of the thesis really didn't matter. I remember well the gist of his advice:

> *Don't try to set the world on fire with your Master's or PhD thesis research and instead focus on getting your "union card" (a completed PhD) as soon as possible. Then get appointed to a university as a faculty member. That's the* **time to start to set the world on fire.**

I liked and accepted his advice. I realized that to get a PhD degree in physiological psychology would require changing universities; the only physiological psychologist at Cornell at the time had little interest in cortical function and was only marginally interested in research. However, rather than waste the year before re-starting a graduate program elsewhere, as I had initially discussed with Dr. Hebb, I decided to work with the Cornell physiological psychologist on a Master's thesis project that fit with his area of interest.

When I returned to Ithaca after the holiday, I reached out to the physiological psychologist. He was delighted with my decision to work with him on a thesis project that would be related to the function of the hippocampus (part of the brain) in rats. My project was approved. Once it was underway, I proceeded to prepare applications to five universities for admission to their PhD physiological psychology programs conditional upon completion of my master's degree. I would start a new program of studies in September 1966. This was an unexpected but not unwelcomed change in plan from my time at DuPont. But first I had to complete my thesis research and then successfully pass my oral examination.

I will always remember that examination. I had been rushing to meet the various submission and documentation deadlines and, having stayed up stayed up late the previous few nights getting prepared for the oral examination, I was tired. I woke up on the morning of the exam with loud banging on my residence door. A fellow student was shouting that my examination committee was waiting for me in the psychology department meeting room. I don't think I have ever moved as fast to throw on some clothes and run the roughly 400 metres from Sage Hall to the psychology department. Although I was feeling rushed, was out of breath, and still had uncombed hair, the exam went beautifully. Everything I had prepared the previous night came to me without hesitation, and I was able to answer the questions remarkably fluently and to actually engage in a discussion of the work without much stuttering. It may have been due to the preparation and my immersion in the work for the previous months. But it may also have been due to the fact that the rush to the examination room had totally distracted me from the usual sense of impending loss of control. The whole experience gave me hope that the prayers of my youth were being answered. If they were, I realized I needed to prepare myself for a life of rushing around distracted. I could live with that if that was what it would take to free myself from stuttering!

* * * * * * * *

Effective that fall, I was accepted for admission to the Ph.D. program at Pennsylvania State University in State College, Pennsylvania, a town located in the dead centre of the state. Penn State had a large and well-known psychology department that offered both research and applied/professional programs. In the early 1960s, the university opened an Animal Behavior Research Lab located on the fringes of the campus. Its director was Dr. J. M. Warren, a senior professor of psychology who was to become my research supervisor.

As with most graduate students at the time, I was offered a teaching assistantship (TA), and my job was to lead small seminar/problem-solving sections for students enrolled in a required undergraduate statistics course. Since I had held the Woodrow Wilson fellowship at Cornell, my TA duties at Penn State constituted my first real experience with university classroom teaching. Fortunately, teaching statistics made extensive use of the blackboard, which was similar enough to a flipchart. I found that if I was writing on the blackboard as I spoke (combined, as I now suspect, with bouncing), my fluency was good enough to get by reasonably well. However, it was evident that I stuttered, and later in the year the professor with responsibility for the course suggested I look into speech therapy in the university's speech clinic. That was the first time anyone had seriously suggested that therapy might help me. More on that later.

Dr. Warren had a number of research areas of interest, including learning theory and the cerebral cortex processes underlying perception and learning in animals (principally cats and rhesus monkeys). Much of the research was on frontal lobe function, and indeed, Dr. Warren had recently co-edited and published an important and influential book of conference proceedings called *Frontal Granular Cortex and Behavior* (Warren & Akert, 1964). The Acquired Brain Injury Outreach Service (ABIOS) of Queensland Health, Australia, characterizes frontal lobe function succinctly as follows:

> "The frontal lobes are important for voluntary movement, expressive language and for managing higher level executive functions. Executive functions refer to a collection of cognitive skills including the capacity to plan, organise, initiate, self-monitor and control one's responses in order to achieve a goal. The frontal lobes are considered our behavioural and emotional control centre and home to our personality."

As I came to realize many years later in a different context, parts of the frontal lobes are an obvious place to look for neurological anomalies that could result in the speech anomalies associated with stuttering. But at that time, I only thought about stuttering when I had to, and that was when I was stuttering or about the speak. At other times, I just tried to blot it out. As it turned out, learning about frontal lobe function under Dr. Warren was a perfect prelude to understanding many years later something of the brain mechanisms associated with stuttering. That said, my own thesis research at Penn State was not concerned directly with frontal lobe function but with exploring in cats the possibility of functional hemispheric asymmetries which are so evident in human split-brain patients.

At this point in my journey, I began to work with a young new faculty colleague of Dr. Warren's in the Animal Behaviour Lab, Dr. Paul Cornwell. Not only was Paul an outstanding research mentor for me, but he also provided a wonderful model of how to teach effectively in a classroom. Although he did not make use of flipcharts, he taught from the blackboard with key words written everywhere, arrows connecting words and ideas, diagrams connected to words, etc. He became a role model, and I practiced his energetic teaching style as best I could in my TA duties. For many years after, when I had a presentation to make or teach a class, I tried to emulate his style. But of course, I added one feature of my own, "bouncing," which at the time I was not fully aware of doing. I still stuttered but, provided I was well prepared and had a blackboard, I could bounce through a presentation. (Just to be clear, I characterize bouncing as repetitions of initial sounds, and so although a lot of repetitions were in my speech, the initial sounds, words, and sentences flowed, but there were few blockages). However, I was still burdened as always with that sense of impending loss of control and with the anxiety it generated about speaking. After some time, it became clear that simply emulating Paul Cornwell's enthusiastic and high energy teaching style, even with a bounce, was not going to be the answer to my stuttering.

My research, which on a day-to-day basis was being supervised by Paul, focused on whether, as in human split-brain patients, there might be evidence of functional hemispheric asymmetries in non-human subjects, specifically cats, whose hemispheres had been surgically separated. The significance of the Penn State research period for this story about stuttering lies far less in the details and findings of this research (Webster, 1972) as in the fact that the work required and encouraged me to immerse myself in the research literature on hemisphere lateralization and, more generally, human neuropsychology and cognitive neuroscience. This prepared me well for my later work involving stuttering. I also became particularly interested in thinking about what the evolutionary significance might be of hemisphere asymmetry—what selective advantage an asymmetrical brain might confer upon a species, human or non-human. I particularly enjoyed preparing and delivering a paper on this subject focusing on territoriality and its possible relationship to the evolution of brain asymmetry (Webster, 1977). As I will return to later in a Reflection Note in chapter 6, the anomalies in brain organization in people who stutter that will have been discussed at that point, could underlie other qualities or attributes in addition to stuttering.

All the while, my stuttering continued despite best efforts, and I was still muddling through. In informal and casual conversations, my speech was up and down but generally somewhat up, but the sense of impending loss of control was almost always with me and led me to hold back and avoid asking questions or making comments or engaging in new conversation whenever I could. Stuttering was most pronounced in conversations with authority figures like professors or the department chair. And the emotions associated with stuttering remained, like the feelings of frustration around the moment-to-moment and situation-to-situation variations in stuttering severity. Accordingly, I decided it was time to accept my professor's advice, mentioned earlier, to consider stuttering therapy offered at the university's speech clinic in the School of Communication Sciences and Disorders. Like speech clinics at other universities, this one provided graduate students in speech-language pathology with opportunities to see clients in a supervised environment. I was hopeful that relief might in fact be found through this route.

When I explained to the student clinician on the reception desk why I was there, I was asked to stick out my tongue, following which I was told that it looked normal. He told me that my stuttering did not seem too bad, and expressed the opinion that nothing could or should be done. I should just live with it. And that was the end of that! My father's words about the futility of stuttering treatment had always echoed in my mind whenever I wondered about treatment. This student-clinician's comment just confirmed my father's opinion that "speech therapy doesn't work." Some years later, I came to see that there is in fact effective speech therapy, but it was not to be found in that student clinic. I would have to wait to see examples of better and more effective treatment options involving speech-language pathologists who specialize in stuttering treatment.

By my second year at Penn State, I had begun to feel quite lonely. I felt isolated from my family because I seldom used a phone to call them, and when I did call, I just wanted to minimize speaking because of the effort. In fact, I seldom used the phone for any purpose and did not even have one in my apartment. In retrospect I am sorry that was how things were. I'm sure my parents would have loved to have heard from me other than for the few days once or twice a year when I made the twelve-hour drive home for a brief visit. The loneliness of this time coincided with two ultimately impactful experiences about stuttering.

Diet-induced Fluency

The few students and research assistants whom I knew were interested in regularly drinking in the evening at the local pub. Feeling lonely, it was easy for me to slip into the role of the passive listener of drunken student philosophizing. I was drinking and smoking more and gaining excess weight in the process. I started to find my clothes didn't really fit any longer, and I didn't have enough money to buy new ones. It was time for some lifestyle changes. And so, I started with a weight loss diet.

I had found a book in the local convenience store that described a low carbohydrate and high protein weight-loss diet, not dissimilar to the current day Atkin's diet or a Keto diet. I was inspired by the book and proceeded to follow the steps, which included eliminating alcohol. It was effective, at least in the short term. By the end of the first month, I had lost twenty-five pounds, was feeling better than I had for a long time, and my clothes again fit. But what truly astonished me was that my stuttering had essentially stopped!

I still remember well my disbelief that I was speaking so fluently and had lost much of the sense of impending loss of control. My professors also noted this change in my speech. However, neither my low carbohydrate diet nor alcohol abstinence lasted, nor did the speech improvement. As I was focusing on getting my doctoral research underway, the diet eased off, beer and snack consumption slowly resumed, and my stuttering returned. But at that point in my studies, I didn't see stuttering to be a "big problem."

I was working mainly on my own, and I was willing to tolerate some stuttering in exchange for returning to the pub, being with others, drinking beer, and eating corn chips. I had no difficulty finding rationalizations that were convincing to me.

It took another decade of stuttering and slow weight gain for me to re-experience "diet-induced fluency" but when I did, I responded to it in a very different manner. More on this in chapter 4.

The Support of Faith

At some point in 1967 or early 1968, I had the experience that my childhood prayers for divine intervention, discussed in chapter 1, were being answered.

Shortly after I had turned out the light one night in my basement apartment in State College, I became acutely aware of a clear white and brightly radiating object or form in the far corner of the room. The light had an elongated humanoid-like size and shape but with no specific features I could discern. I truly felt at that moment that I was in the presence of God or the Holy Spirit or an angel made manifest. The form simply radiated a white light, and I remember thinking the light didn't seem to illuminate the room or create shadows; it was just bright and self-contained. Although I recall nothing actually being spoken out loud, I nonetheless very much "heard" the form conveying to me in a reassuring way that I would find peace with myself and with others about my stuttering, and I should not worry about stuttering. I interpreted some of what was being "said" to mean that I would come to view my stuttering as something about me that would contribute meaning to my life and there was no need to be dismayed by it. And then, after a short time, the light and form slowly faded away leaving the room in darkness. I did not get out of bed, but simply lay still, soaking up what I had just experienced. I was not frightened; in fact, I felt in awe; I felt calm; and I felt an exquisitely deep sense of peace and reassurance. Was this the "cure" for which I had prayed for so many years? If so, it was not quite what I had expected and hoped for as a response.

I have reflected on this experience many times over the subsequent years. At the time, it must have been at least two years since I had last prayed for relief from stuttering, and I have no recollection of having been unusually preoccupied with my speech at the time. Just more of the same stuttering, holding back, and as I anticipated speaking situations, the usual sense of impending loss of control. Based on the light and lack of shadow patterns, I doubted I had experienced through my senses something that was actually occurring physically in the room. I also doubted that this was merely a simple hallucination or a false perception of objects in the room. I had never taken drugs. I had not been drinking in recent days. I was not particularly tired. I had no fever or illness. I had not experienced anything like this before. Instead, I came to view this "visitation" as being a spiritual occurrence, one that was generated and guided by the spiritual force I had sensed in the room at the time, and one that was directly influencing my brain activity and, through that, my thought processes and perceptions. This, of course, raised many further questions for me. For example, if there was a spiritual force underlying this experience, had subsequent (or earlier) experiences and "choices" in my life been influenced or guided by this Holy Spirit or angel or spiritual force, unconsciously on my part? Is that why and how I ended up spending so much of my subsequent years learning about stuttering and its management, and through those discoveries, found peace and reassurance as promised? Was it destiny or merely chance that so many of the opportunities that gave direction to my journey were so closely aligned temporally with my readiness to respond positively to them? These are unanswerable questions, but that does not detract from the impact of the experience on me.

Regardless of its source or cause, the experience brought me at the time a real sense of peace about my stuttering. I still stuttered, sometimes very severely; I still had a sense of impending loss of control at the prospect of having to speak; I still held back; however, I no longer felt as angry or discouraged about my speech and its potential negative impact on my future. From time to time over the subsequent years, I felt that this angel continued to watch over me, a sense that would give me solace and hope and patience with myself and my speech. In more recent years, I developed a better appreciation of the many positive things in my life that came about directly or indirectly by my being a person who stutters. Looking back, I wouldn't change a thing about my life, including, believe it or not, my stuttering.

* * * * * * * *

It was nearly time to "start to set the world on fire" as Dr. Hebb had suggested. As my doctoral program was nearing completion, I was anxious to return to Canada and start an academic position. I was tired of being poor and, even though I knew I still had a lot to learn, tired of being a student. So, I decided to apply to several Canadian universities for an assistant professor position in psychology.

Four of the universities to which I had applied expressed interest in meeting with me and having me make a presentation about my research interests. I was fortunate because at that particular time there was a glut of faculty positions open in psychology, a situation that would change dramatically within two years when the doors slammed shut on faculty appointments everywhere and in most discipline for many years after. My presentations were frankly poor. I still remember that my speech was not very fluent, I felt hung over at one presentation, and I felt self-conscious and uncomfortable at others. Perhaps I was still doubtful that someone who stutters really could be a university professor and all that entails. But fortunately for me the bar for hiring was low that year. I was offered positions at three universities. I decided to accept the offer from Carleton University in Ottawa, Ontario, to start in July, 1969.

A good choice, it turned out, because that was where my research on brain mechanisms underlying stuttering would eventually be inspired and carried out.

PART II

Time to Set the World on Fire

CHAPTER 4

My World as a Young and New Professor Who Stuttered

I t was a good time both personally and professionally to be at Carleton University. With roughly 35 full-time faculty members, the relatively young department was developing a good reputation for its undergraduate teaching. The graduate programs were still new and evolving in promising ways, and covered the areas of developmental psychology, social psychology, physiological psychology, and learning/cognitive psychology. New faculty members were given great latitude and support to pursue their individual research and teaching interests, which was one of the reasons I was attracted to Carleton in the first place.

In my initial job interview at Carleton, I had committed to continue my research on hemisphere asymmetries in animals. The department gave me essentially carte blanche to order the equipment and supplies I would need upon my arrival. I was well treated, but like many new faculty members, I started to struggle almost immediately due to the need to juggle competing personal and professional priorities.

Complicating matters, I had not actually completed my PhD thesis when my appointment took effect in July 1969. I estimated that I had three weeks of work left to complete the final thesis preparation. What with moving to Ottawa, getting my courses organized (and that included filling in many knowledge gaps), applying for an operating research grant, ordering supplies for my lab, learning new material that had to be incorporated into my courses, being newly married with a wife who was expecting, and experiencing six or eight weeks of brain fog associated with having stopped cigarette smoking in early 1970, it took 8 months to complete the estimated three weeks remaining on the thesis and oral defence.

If I was to be reasonably fluent, give credible lectures, and lead discussions in my classes, all of which were important to me, I needed to do a great deal of preparation. That usually included essentially writing a script for each class to which I could refer as needed. At that time, as I have alluded to earlier, because so much of my attention while lecturing was focused on my speech and that sense of impending loss of control, I needed to have both the "what" and the "how" of my classes well laid out. Compounding the issue of the time required to prepare for classroom teaching was my having agreed with the department to develop and, starting in my third year, to teach a new hands-on research methods laboratory course in physiological psychology. Planning the course and its logistics was demanding and offering such a course in fact required writing a textbook (Webster, 1975). Although actually teaching the new course was less onerous with respect to speaking than a regular lecture course would be, it meant substantially more hours per week of student contact. Research ethics issues about using live animals for undergraduate teaching were beginning to emerge as problematic at this time, and so the course did not continue to be offered after four or five years.

Shortly after my arrival at Carleton, I had applied for and received a research grant from the National Research Council (soon to become the Natural Sciences and Engineering Research Council) but it was not sufficient for me to hire a research assistant to assist meaningfully with the behavioral testing of the cats. It started to become apparent that the research program I had naïvely envisaged in my interview might not be feasible to carry out at this stage of my career. I found that I could not do both the class preparation and teaching, on the one hand, and the animal testing on the other, and so testing was compromised. Haphazard research is never good research, and for me there was an ethical issue about using animals (or humans) for research when the benefits of that research are at best suspect. I also began to question whether the benefits of the planned research, no matter how well done, would be sufficient to justify the highly invasive surgical procedures and resulting discomfort for the animals.

This question of research ethics had never arisen at Penn State. After arriving at Carleton, I was influenced by a consideration of the guidelines for the ethical use of animals in teaching and research recently promulgated at the time by the Canadian Council on Animal Care. I came to recognize and acknowledge that the cats, although legally acquired from a commercial firm in Quebec, had probably been house pets, possibly even cat-napped off the street. On a personal level, I was increasingly troubled about the probable origins of the animals and the procedures to be used in the planned research program.

During the rest of that first decade at Carleton, my research activities never achieved focus and were, frankly, a hodgepodge of initiatives. I was hardly "setting the world on fire" as Dr. Hebb said I should, but I was nonetheless learning a lot about being an academic. On the research front, I returned briefly to a previous interest at Penn State on paw preferences in animals (Warren et al., 1972) and I published two research articles with students on this subject (Martin & Webster, 1974; Webster & Shoup, 1975). I also tried to modify the hemisphere asymmetry research in cats so it would involve less invasive procedures than cutting the corpus callosum and optic chiasm. However, studying hemispheric engagement in behaviour by recording and analyzing EEG signals from the brain (Brito & Webster, 1979) did not really solve the ethics problem nor the time problem, and the initial results were not particularly encouraging. I was also struggling with philosophy of science type questions related to how to conceptualize the "functions of the brain" in the context of behavior and psychological processes (Webster, 1973). This all led to my starting to study aspects of functional hemisphere asymmetries in humans using non-invasive techniques (e.g., Webster & Thurber, 1978) like those to which I was originally introduced through the *Interhemispheric Relations and Cerebral Dominance* book (Mountcastle, 1962).

But as I came to realize and finally accept near the end of that initial decade, the real issue underlying the lack of research focus was that I was on a slippery slope towards alcoholism. My consumption had been increasing as a way of responding to the stresses associated with constant speaking demands but, ironically, alcohol actually made speaking even more difficult. I felt that a drink might relax me, but the numbing did not translate into better speech nor a reduced sense of impending loss of control. I remember well many professional and social functions at which, after a couple of drinks (or more, if I am to be honest), my speech blockages got so severe I could not engage in conversation at all.

At some point in the latter half of the 1970s, I decided that I had to stop drinking entirely and get myself into better physical and psychological shape. My father had been a man of his times and, like many of his contemporaries, not only worked long hours, but smoked heavily and drank a lot. He was not a good role model, and I knew that a path of "liquid lunches" was not one I wanted to follow. I had stopped smoking shortly after I arrived at Carleton, and I was now determined to cut out alcohol as well. After a number of false starts, I returned to the same weight-loss diet I had been on ten years earlier while a student: low carbohydrate (including no alcohol) and high protein. This time I lost nearly thirty pounds in about forty-five days. As before when I was at Penn State, I didn't want to stop the diet because my speech had improved so much. At the end of the active dieting, I did not resume drinking as I had done when I had been a student. And I became much more engaged with physical fitness activities like swimming and bicycling. I experienced one brief relapse but the impact of that on my speech provided a sharp reminder of why alcohol had to go permanently. Despite the social pressure in the university environment to drink, I persevered with abstinence, and I continue that today. One of my better choices.

This improvement in my speech with the dieting and abstinence occurred at a propitious time. By the late-1970s the psychology department at Carleton had become dysfunctional due to faculty tensions and conflict. It was time to elect a new department chair. For some reason, despite my speech difficulties, I seem to have been looked upon as someone who might be able to lead the department, maintain its credibility, and have influence with the university administration—either that or else I was seen to be a "push-over" who would do the administrative paper-work and leave faculty members alone. Either way, I suspect I was seen as being the only person whose arm could be twisted to do what was generally seen to be a thankless job. Having grown up in an academic family and having developed a deep respect and fondness for the concept of a university, I didn't happen to share that "thankless job" perspective on the chair position. I had seen at Carleton, as well as through my father's stories about McGill and elsewhere, that department chairs can and do make a real difference to a department and the wellbeing of students and faculty colleagues. Also, although I had some difficulty admitting it to myself, I was beginning to think that I could make a greater contribution to the university, the department, and the discipline of psychology by supporting and facilitating the research and scholarship of my colleagues rather than through my own limited research endeavours. And so, when unanimous support was offered by my colleagues for me to become department chair, I felt honoured and, without thinking too much about the matter, I agreed.

What had I done? I had thrust myself into a position that required speaking in every kind of situation I found difficult: making phone calls to strangers; answering the phone; introducing myself; chairing meetings large and small; presenting the curriculum vitae of faculty colleagues to the Faculty tenure and promotion committee; dealing with hostile students and parents with complaints; dealing with allegations of improper behaviour by someone or other; attending university social events; speaking off the cuff at public events; recommending faculty for salary adjustments, and more.

All I could do about my speech when I couldn't avoid speaking was to build upon the few techniques or tricks that seemed to have helped me in the past: detailed preparation, so I did not have to both formulate what needed to be said and to figure out how to say it; using a flipchart or white board when presenting to the faculty so I could both write and talk together; emulating Paul Cornwell's high energy teaching style whenever it was appropriate and might work; avoiding situations for as long as possible whenever I could; using bouncing to keep the flow of speech moving; relying more on writing detailed notes which I could fall back on if necessary; writing memos rather than phoning or talking face to face; becoming more of an active listener so I was not so preoccupied with that sense of impending loss of control. But it was all still very much a matter of muddling through.

And while these new responsibilities that involved speaking made my life more difficult and stressful, they also released me from most of my formal classroom teaching duties. As department chair, I received a significantly reduced classroom teaching load, and this made my life easier and less stressful (probably for the students too). I welcomed the new experiences and new issues, and I enjoyed being involved in decision-making at the department and Faculty levels. As department chair, I was also provided with university research funds sufficient to augment my grant so I could hire a part-time research assistant to help me with my research (although by this time I had abandoned my work with cats). The change in roles also encouraged me to avoid all alcohol, limit other carbohydrates, and swim and bicycle regularly. I was desperate to do all I could to be as fluent as possible, and drinking beer and engaging in emotional eating did not help. Fear of shame and humiliation can be a great motivator.

At about the time I had been appointed as department chair, I was invited to participate in a neuropsychology conference at Oxford University. When I arrived at the London airport, I ran into an old friend whom I had met some years earlier at Penn State and with whom I had stayed in occasional contact. He, too, was on his way to Oxford for the conference. As we rode on the bus together, the subject turned to my stuttering, and I told him about my experience with dieting and the improved speech I had been experiencing.

We both began to speculate on what might underlie the diet effect on my speech (assuming it was real). My friend immediately looked to neurotransmitter explanations. Were the speech improvements related to neurochemical changes resulting from reduced alcohol consumption, reduced carbohydrate consumption, including sugar, or to increased protein consumption? Was more exercise a factor? Or was I just feeling better, healthier, and more in control of life generally? Of course, we couldn't answer these questions because so little was known (by us, at least) about the brain mechanisms underlying stuttering. That casual bus conversation would provide me shortly with a whole new thrust to my research aspirations which led ultimately to my understanding of much of the neuropsychological basis of my stuttering.

It seemed evident that the key initial questions that I needed to answer were the most basic: What is different about the brain of the person who stutters? What underlies the variation in stuttering severity across time and situations? My initial thoughts were that I might be able to pursue those questions by building on my theoretical, conceptual, and methodological background in neuropsychology. But I would first need to immerse myself in the research literature on stuttering. I realized that only after those two initial questions had been answered would I be in a position to explore how the diet might have had its effects (either centrally or peripherally) on my speech.

As I flew home to Canada, I felt that I finally had some real direction for my future research efforts. Over the previous fifteen-year period, my interests had wandered, for good and bad. I had moved from a career trajectory involving advertising and marketing research to one focused on social psychology and then neuroscience. I had changed universities. I had completed graduate degrees in different subject areas. I had developed a good command of the research literature on cortical function and hemisphere asymmetries (human and non-human). I had published several articles and book chapters on disparate topics, and a textbook on research methods. I had also taken first steps into university administration and a leadership role as department chair. And now I would become immersed with the research and clinical literature in a whole new area for me, stuttering. I would shortly become involved with a clinical stuttering treatment program and its clients through which I would acquire a whole new perspective on stuttering and on people who stutter.

What a privileged situation I was in to have the flexibility to be able to so readily pursue new academic interests. Now it was time to follow my calling and hopefully set the world on fire through three concurrent but relatively independent tracks:

- My laboratory research on brain mechanisms and stuttering that flowed from the experience I had going to Oxford. This will be discussed in chapters 5 and 6.
- The volunteer experiences I had over several years working in a clinical context with speech-language pathologists and with people who stutter. This will be discussed in chapter 7.
- My academic leadership and administrative work, first as a department chair at Carleton University and then followed by my role as a dean at two other universities and a brief interlude as director of a professional school in speech-language pathology and audiology. These roles and the speech demands associated with each will all be discussed in chapter 8.

These tracks ran in parallel yet, despite being separate, they did influence one another. As I learned new things in each track, they shaped my view of how I might approach the management of my stuttering. Chapter 9 brings together and integrates what I learned from these three tracks and suggests and provides a rationale for some strategies for managing stuttering.

CHAPTER 5

The Brain of the Person Who Stutters: Speech Motor Control

F ollowing the bus trip to the Oxford conference, the directions for my future had suddenly become clearer and I began to realize the calling that awaited me. To reiterate, the two key initial questions that would guide my research were as follows:

> What is different about the brain of the person who stutters compared to the brain of the person who does not stutter?

> What underlies the variation in stuttering severity across time and situations? Or, expressed in a different way, what happens in the brains of people who stutter as they go from fluent speech to periods of disfluent speech and back to fluent speech?

That encounter constituted another unpredicted and defining twist in my life journey. I now realize that my father's dismissal of the efficacy of speech therapy for stuttering had led me to assume implicitly that stuttering was forever. It started to dawn on me that once I understood more about the neurological underpinnings of stuttering, I might not feel or be as helpless as I had thought about living with a stutter. Through my teaching of physiological psychology at Carleton, I was quite familiar of the concept of neuroplasticity and how our brain organization and activity can be altered but, ironically and as bizarre as it really is, it hadn't occurred to me that alterations might apply in the stuttering context.

Upon my return home, I started a detailed study of the research literature on stuttering. The previous 20 years, the 1960s and 1970s, had seen a growing body of research publications in speech-language pathology and neuropsychology that pointed to a significant role for biological factors underlying stuttering. Noteworthy in this regard were studies of genetic factors in stuttering (Howie, 1981; Kidd, 1984) and brain mechanisms.

The concept of a central nervous system basis to stuttering was not new at that time. In fact, one model of stuttering, which continued to influence contemporary thought in the 1970s, had been proposed nearly a century ago by Dr. Samuel Orton, a neurologist, and Dr. Lee Edward Travis, a psychologist and speech-language pathologist. It held that stuttering is due to an anomaly or peculiarity in interhemispheric relations. More specifically, Orton (1928) and Travis (1931, 1978) argued that, in contrast to the fluent speaker whose speech and language processes are controlled by the left hemisphere, the person who stutters has centres for speech control in both hemispheres rather than just one. According to their model, which is illustrated conceptually in figure 1, having these bilateral neural mechanisms results in two sets of commands being sent to the speech musculature, commands which if even slightly out of synchrony would result in discoordination—and that is stuttering.

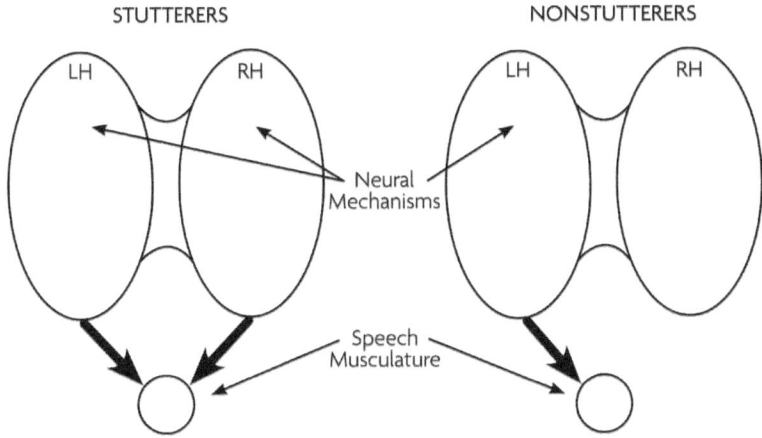

Figure 1. Schematic diagram of the Orton/Travis model of stuttering.
(LH=left hemisphere; RH=right hemisphere).

Before examining this model in detail, some comments are required about the pattern of lateralization found in the normal human brain.

Two somewhat interchangeable terms often used to describe inter-hemispheric relations in human brain organization are **lateralization** and **hemisphere specialization**. These terms refer to the fact that, although the two hemispheres are anatomically similar in size and shape, certain cognitive and behavioural functions are mediated primarily by one or the other hemisphere. In this sense, the functions are said to be **lateralized**. **Hemisphere specialization** refers to the particular functions in a lateralized brain. Among the best documented of these functions relates to speech and language, mediated mainly by the left hemisphere in most individuals. As has been known for well over a century (Young, 1970), damage to the left hemisphere can result in changes in speech and language not found following comparable damage to the right hemisphere. Right hemisphere damage has its own unique effects.

As discussed in chapter 3, the complementary nature of hemisphere specialization had been, in my view and at that time, most dramatically demonstrated in those individual patients with intractable epilepsy who had the corpus callosum sectioned in the midline (Sperry, 1974). The rationale for the surgery was to limit the spread of seizures from one hemisphere to the other. There are remarkably few obvious negative consequences of this procedure. Despite the cerebral hemispheres having been surgically separated, a unity of conscious awareness continues. However, with special testing methods, it becomes clear that patients can talk only about information directed to the left hemisphere. Although there may have been some debate about the capacity of the right hemisphere to process **language** in these split-brain cases (Gazzaniga, 1983; Zaidel, 1983) and in neurologically normal people (Perecman, 1983; Searleman, 1977), there is little debate about **speech**. Almost always, it is a left hemisphere function.

In contrast, tasks that involve **visuo-constructional** skills (Young & Ratcliff, 1984), such as arranging blocks in certain spatial configurations, are far better performed when the split-brain person is using the left hand (controlled by the right hemisphere) rather than the right hand (controlled by the left hemisphere). Emerging out of this research literature is a first generalization about human brain organization:

> *The two cerebral hemispheres in humans are specialized for different forms of cognitive processing. In most people, the left hemisphere is the one specialized for speech and language functions, and the right hemisphere for visuo-spatial functions, among other things.*

Contrary to some out-dated but persisting popular notions of cerebral dominance, this generalization applies to right-handers and most left-handers. This is evident in the results of the assessment of hemisphere specialization for speech, language, and memory using what is called the Wada test, named after the neurologist Juhn Wada who developed it. A short acting anesthetic is infused into one carotid artery and then, later, into the other. In most people, infusions into the left carotid artery, which supplies blood primarily to the left hemisphere, result in a brief speech cessation, whereas infusions into the right carotid artery leave speech intact. Virtually all right-handers demonstrate evidence of left hemisphere dominance for speech and language. Although less predictable, the majority of left-handers do as well (Milner, Branch, & Rasmussen, 1966).

Although the two cerebral hemispheres are of similar size and shape, a number of consistent anatomical asymmetries between the hemispheres probably underlie these functional asymmetries. Without going into detail, one major area of anatomical asymmetry is the planum temporale, located on the upper posterior surface of the temporal lobe. In their classic paper, Geschwind and Levitsky (1968) reported that in about two-thirds of 100 brains examined, the planum temporale was larger in the left hemisphere than in the right. It was larger on the right side in about ten percent of the brains and was of similar size in the two hemispheres in the remaining twenty-five percent. The planum temporale is part of the classical posterior language area, referred to as Wernicke's area (Galaburda et al., 1978). Damage to this area has long been known to result in **receptive aphasia**, meaning difficulties in language comprehension. Anatomical asymmetries have also been identified in Broca's area (Albanese et al., 1989; Foundas et al., 1995; Hayes & Lewis, 1985), an anterior area which, if damaged, usually results in speech production difficulties called **expressive aphasia**.

This research all leads to a second generalization about human brain organization:

> *Although the two hemispheres are of the same general size and shape, a number of consistent anatomical asymmetries are generally thought to underlie the functional asymmetries in speech and language processing in fluent speakers.*

The 1960s and 1970s saw the development of clinical and experimental neuropsychological methods used in the assessment and study of hemisphere specialization. These were many of the same methods to which I had been introduced in my early days as a graduate student at Cornell when reading *Interhemispheric Relations and Cerebral Dominance* (Mountcastle, 1962). The research included, for example, dichotic listening and visual half-field studies of neurologically intact research participants. These methods will be discussed in more detail later in the context of research with people who stutter. Briefly, however, dichotic listening involves a person listening to competing **verbal** messages going to the two ears separately through earphones, and usually the message directed to the right ear is better attended to and recalled than the message directed to the left ear. This is similar to the presentation of visual information to the right and left visual half-fields separately. Verbal information directed to the right visual half-field is processed more efficiently than information to the left half-field. At that time, it was generally accepted that these perceptual asymmetries reflect neurological asymmetries, but contemporary thinking that I will discuss in chapter 6 also places emphasis also on attentional factors in the context of hemisphere activation.

What is Meant by "Visual Half-Fields"

If you stare straight ahead, everything you can see to the right of your fixation point is said to be in the right visual half-field of each eye, and everything you can see to the left of the fixation point is in the left visual half-field of each eye. Because of the organization of the optic nerve and optic tract, the right visual half-fields of the two eyes project directly to the left hemisphere and the left visual half-fields project directly to the right hemisphere.

These methods, together with the general acceptance of these first two generalizations of brain organization, made the Orton (1928) and Travis (1931) model the focus of considerable research effort during the 1970s related to stuttering. The literature I was reviewing contained a good number of comparisons of people who stutter with people who do not stutter. It is not my intention to summarize or review that literature except to say that the pattern of data bearing on the Orton (1928) and Travis (1931) model was conflicting and inconclusive. However, it was consistent with the general idea that people who stutter, or some subgroup of people who stutter, have some form of aberration or peculiarity or anomaly in **interhemispheric relations**. Unfortunately, little emerged from the literature as to the nature of the anomaly.

I decided at that time that my research program would focus initially on developing and testing neuropsychological models of potential forms of anomalous interhemispheric relations in people who stutter, starting with the Orton and Travis model.

In my research, I did not study speech per se nor use brain imaging technology like positron emission tomography (PET scans) or functional magnetic resonance imaging (fMRI). Instead, my research was based on the theory and methods of experimental neuropsychology to make inferences about brain organization related to speech based on differences between people who stutter and those who do not with respect to unimanual and bimanual motor movement control. A large body of research (Kimura, 1982, 1993; Goodale, 1988; Mateer, 1983; Ojemann, 1983; Roland, 1985; Roland et al., 1980) had indicated that the neural mechanisms for the control of movement of the hands and fingers overlap those that control speech. Accordingly, my basic assumption was that as I came to understand possible anomalies in the control of the **fingers and hands** in people who stutter, I would come to understand something of the anomalies in their **speech** motor movement control.

Using this framework to test the Orton and Travis model, and with the assistance of my incredible research assistant, Joanne Hakkaku, my initial study (Webster, 1985) built upon the observation that most people, both right- and left-handed, tap the fingers of the right hand faster and more accurately than the fingers of the left-hand (Denkla, 1983; Peters, 1980; Todor & Kyrie, 1980). This effect is apparent with tapping a single finger repeatedly, as well as with sequential finger tapping in which research participants are asked to tap telegraph keys repeatedly in a particular order using their four fingers, as in playing a musical instrument. The usual interpretation of the right-hand advantage (Kinsbourne & McMurray, 1975; Lomas & Kimura, 1976; Peters, 1980; Wolff, Hurwitz & Moss, 1977) was that the right hand has direct access to the left hemisphere specialized mechanisms for movement sequencing and fine motor control. In contrast, the motor cortex controlling the left hand has access to these commands only after they have crossed to the right hemisphere. The prediction under the Orton and Travis model was that, if stutterers have bilateral speech (and other) motor control mechanisms, they should also have bilateral control of other fine motor movements. Accordingly, under the model, stutterers should **not** show a right-hand advantage in finger tapping; fingers of the two hands should show similar tapping performance.

Our research participants in this and most other studies of mine were adults recruited from the community at large and from the university using newspaper advertisements. Other participants were volunteers from the

Stuttering Treatment Program of the Royal Ottawa Rehabilitation Centre (now called the Ottawa Hospital Rehabilitation Centre). As I recount in more detail in chapter 7, I had asked the speech-language pathologists at the Centre if they could assist me in recruiting participants from their treatment program for the research, and they agreed. Many of my research studies included only males who stuttered because of their 4:1 prevalence (2:1 in children) in the general population, but in some studies sex and handedness were variables in addition to fluency status.

Introduction to the late Dr. Einer Boberg

At this point, before discussing the research studies themselves, I want to briefly introduce the late Dr. Einer Boberg, an outstanding and accomplished speech-language pathologist who was himself a person who stuttered, specialized in the study of stuttering and its treatment, and was a strong supporter and facilitator of self-help groups. He also played the violin (far better than me). A few of his publications are cited in this book. Dr. Boberg was a professor at the University of Alberta and, together with his colleague, Deborah Kully, founded the Institute for Stuttering Treatment and Research (ISTAR) in 1986. For many years he was a real leader of the international stuttering research community, and he loved bringing people together to discuss research issues. I greatly appreciated how he understood, valued, and encouraged my approach to the basic research questions I was asking, and how much I learned by being included by him in several conferences that he organized on stuttering. I contributed a chapter (Webster, 1993) to his well-known edited book, *Neuropsychology of Stuttering*, and we wrote one paper together (Boberg & Webster, 1990) during his sabbatical leave in Ottawa. From the start, he was a supportive professional friend whose perspective I greatly valued.

The first study was designed to test the Orton/Travis theory of stuttering by using a **repetitive sequential finger tapping** task performed by stutterers and non-stutterers. The apparatus was comprised of four telegraph keys wired individually to different channels of a chart recorder. Participants rested their fingers on the keys, and every time a key was pressed, a pen on the corresponding chart recorder channel would move. This allowed me to measure the timing and sequencing of key presses.

On each fifteen-second trial of this task, the participant was to tap the keys repeatedly in a specified sequence, such as 1-2-3-4 or 3-1-2-4, where 1 indicates the index finger and 4 the little finger. They were instructed to tap each sequence as rapidly and as accurately as possible. Testing of each sequence with each hand was under conditions of both visual guidance on some trials and no visual guidance on others.

Three aspects of tapping performance were measured: 1) the number of correct sequences tapped in each fifteen-second trial, 2) the total number of key presses in each trial, and 3) the number of incorrect responses in each trial. Incorrect responses might have included extra key presses (e.g., 1-2-3-2-4 instead of 1-2-3-4), key presses in incorrect order (e.g., 1-2-4-3 instead of 1-2-3-4), or omissions from the sequence of key depressions (e.g., 1-3-4 instead of 1-2-3-4).

The performance of the two groups, adult stutterers and adult fluent speakers, was almost identical. This result was clearly contrary to the prediction based on the Orton and Travis model. Both groups of participants showed a right-hand advantage. They also showed similar overall rates of tapping indicating that the stutterers were not generally uncoordinated or motorically slow. There was, however, a small but nonetheless reliable difference between the groups in errors, a finding that I will return to shortly.

My interpretation of the data was that there is normal left hemisphere lateralization in people who stutter. This is a conclusion similar to that reached from Wada technique studies which assessed cerebral dominance in people who stutter. As discussed previously, almost all right-handed people and most left-handed people cease speaking briefly after left but not right carotid artery infusions. As described by Andrews, Quinn, and Sorby (1972) and Luessenhop, Boggs, Laborwit, and Walle (1973), people who stutter responded to these left- and right-sided infusions of anesthetic in the same way as did fluent speakers, indicating again a normal pattern of hemisphere specialization for speech. Moore (1993) reported that the electroencephalographic (EEG) recordings from the two hemispheres of stutterers and non-stutterers show no differences during a **resting state**

condition with no speaking. Consistent with these findings, Ingham, Fox, and Ingham (1997) more recently reported no differences in PET scan neuroimages recorded from stutterers and non-stutterers during a **resting state** condition. Ingham et al. (1997) concluded that their findings do not support "suggestions that developmental stuttering is associated with abnormalities of brain blood flow at rest. In other words, their brain physiology is normal [when speech is not being used]" (p. 302). As will be discussed later in chapter 6, the analyses of neuroimages recorded during **speaking tasks** paint a very different picture. Although as we will see shortly, stuttering is associated with anomalous brain activation during speech, it is important for the reader to appreciate that there is no suggestion in any of this research that the person who stutters is brain damaged. We are dealing with a normal brain that, for reasons basically of its "wiring," is functioning in an anomalous fashion when processing speech and language.

These research findings lead me to a generalization about cerebral lateralization related to stuttering:

> *People who stutter have normal left hemisphere lateralization of the neural mechanisms for the control of speech and other forms of sequential motor performance.*

Despite the apparently normal lateralization that was evident in the results of this sequential finger tapping study (Webster, 1985), I began to suspect that the left hemisphere mechanisms in stutterers may not in fact be as **efficient** as they are in fluent speakers. The possibility that the sequential finger tapping task was not sufficiently sensitive to detect group differences was first suggested by the slightly elevated error rate of stutterers on finger tapping, as noted earlier. It was also suggested by the fact that two of eighteen stutterers had been eliminated from the analysis because they were unable to perform the sequential finger-tapping task with any degree of proficiency. And a third concern was that the parallel I was assuming between **repetitive sequential finger-tapping** and the **serially ordered aspects of speech** may have been tenuous. The speech difficulty experienced by most people who stutter is related more to the **initiation** of new utterances than to their **repetition**. This repetition phenomenon is referred to in speech-language pathology as the "adaptation effect" (Bloodstein, 1981): disfluencies decrease as a sentence or phrase is repeated. Perhaps if I had focused more on the **initiation** of finger tapping rather than its continuing **speed and accuracy**, I would have had different findings.

So, I undertook another study (Webster, 1986a) which required the participants to tap on each trial a **new** sequence that had just been demonstrated briefly on a display panel rather than tapping the **same** sequence repeatedly. I called this the **sequence reproduction task**. It was to tell us about the efficiency with which stutterers and non-stutterers can plan and initiate and organize new sequences of motor movements, which would seem to parallel a critical component of speech production. On this task, participants who stuttered were slower and made more errors than fluent controls in reproducing the sequences under both speeded (Webster, 1986a, 1989a) and non-speeded (Webster, 1989b) conditions. Let's look at this in more detail.

The study started with a replication of our findings with the repetitive sequential finger task. I found the same effects described earlier: no difference between the groups in the speed and accuracy of tapping the same sequence repeatedly. It's always good when you can replicate findings with new participants. These same participants, stutterers and non-stutterers, were then tested and compared on the sequence reproduction task.

Each trial of the sequence reproduction task started with the presentation on a visual display panel of a new finger-tap sequence to be performed using the same telegraph key setup used in the repetitive sequence tapping task. Immediately following the presentation on the display, a tone sounded, and the participant was to tap the sequence on the telegraph keys as quickly and as accurately as possible for 5 seconds. Included were all different combinations of four-element sequences (except ones beginning with the little finger) (e.g., 2-3-4-1 or 3-1-4-2) without repeated elements. To introduce unpredictability to the situation, three- and five-element sequences (e.g., 1-3-2, and 1-4-2-1-3, respectively), and four-element sequences with a repeated element (e.g., 2-1-3-1) were interspersed at random among the four-element sequences that were my main interest. Only the data from the four-element sequences without a repeated element were analyzed; the other trials were essentially distractors. In addition to the same measures of response accuracy described earlier in the context of the repetitive sequential finger tapping study, measurements were made of the **response-initiation** times (i.e., the time from the start of the tone to the first key press) and **sequence execution** times (i.e., the time to carry out the first complete sequence). Of particular interest with respect to accuracy was the initial sequence tapped. Two important sets of findings emerged from this study.

- First, participants who stuttered were significantly slower than fluent controls in initiating their responses. They also made more errors in carrying out the first sequence.
- However, once the stutterers got started with a sequence, their performance was just as fast and just as accurate as that of the non-stutterers.

The implication of these data was that people who stutter have difficulty with the **organization and initiation** of new non-speech sequential movements just as they do with the organization and initiation of new speech utterances. We found in a separate study (Webster, 1989b) that even when there was no time pressure, stutterers still made significantly more errors than fluent controls in reproducing the sequences.

These results led directly to the second key question that started this research program, "What changes in the brain of the person who stutters as he/she goes from periods of fluency to periods of disfluency?" The variability in stuttering severity, so characteristic of the disorder and so frustrating for those of us who stutter, implies an underlying mechanism that is **dynamic** rather than one that reflects a **fixed or static** condition. In other words, if stuttering is associated with an inefficient left hemisphere motor sequencing system, something that is variable must be acting on that system to result in the discoordination associated with speech in people who stutter. In a number of experiments, we have explored the possibility that these dynamic processes are ones that involve interference on the left hemisphere system by neural activity in the right hemisphere.

Our initial idea about the nature of the interference is illustrated in the model shown in figure 2. Referred to simply as the Interhemispheric Interference Model, it assumed normal left hemisphere lateralization of speech processes and other fine motor movement in people who stutter. I thought there might be an overflow of right hemisphere activity that produces interference on this left hemisphere motor area, analogous to static on a radio. Such overflow could be due to an **overactivation** of the right hemisphere; or to a problem with the corpus callosum **gating** of neural activity transfer between the hemispheres resulting in crosstalk; or to a heightened **sensitivity** of the left hemisphere motor mechanisms to normal right hemisphere activity; and there are other possibilities. Regardless of the underlying mechanisms, according to this model variations in stuttering severity reflect variations in the impact of neural activity overflow from the right to the left hemisphere.

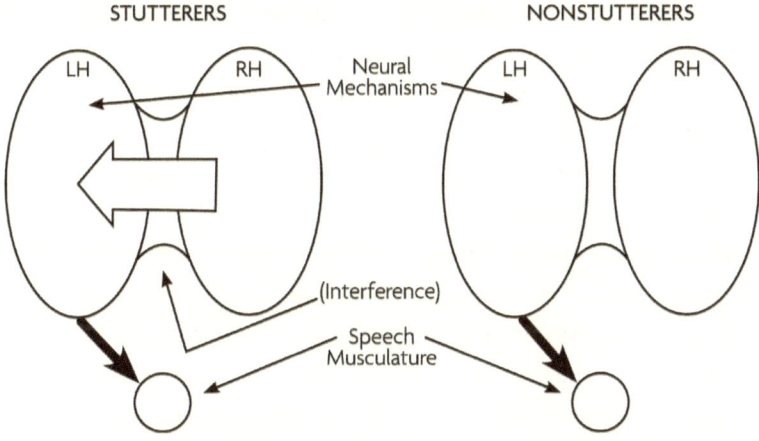

Figure 2. Schematic diagram of the Interhemispheric Interference Model.
(LH=left hemisphere; RH=right hemisphere)

But what evidence is there that right hemisphere activity could be the source (or one of the sources) of interference with the left hemisphere?

At the time of the literature review in 1980, a small but provocative body of research supported the idea that, in contrast to people who are fluent speakers, stutterers engage the right hemisphere when processing speech. For example, instead of showing the usual right listening ear advantage in dichotic listening, people who stutter show little or no difference between the two ears in information recalled. Clearer evidence has been found in the electrophysiological activity recorded from the right and left hemispheres of people who stutter. Not only did people who stutter show anomalous right hemisphere EEG activation during verbal information processing (Boberg et al., 1983, Yeudall et al., 1983; Moore, 1986; Moore & Haynes, 1980), but the pattern was reported to shift toward the more normal pattern of left hemisphere activation following successful stuttering therapy (Boberg et al., 1983).

The pattern of results in these studies could be interpreted as indicating bilateral speech control as proposed by Orton and Travis. However, as discussed earlier, the Wada testing (Andrews et al., 1972; Luessenhop et al., 1973) and the PET scan analysis of the brains of people who stutter under resting conditions (Ingham et al., 1997) make that unlikely. More likely it could mean that the right hemisphere, lacking the specialized neural systems required for efficient and effective verbal processing, becomes engaged during speaking for **non-linguistic** reasons. On possible reason could be related to the prosodic aspects of speech (meaning "relating to the rhythm and intonation of language"); another might be the emotional or fear- and anxiety-related aspects of oral communication for stutterers. This idea will be returned to later in the chapter.

First, to test the model in figure 2, I took advantage of the fact that each hemisphere controls the opposite hand, and we developed experimental analogues of the old parlor game of rubbing your stomach and patting your head at the same time. If there is an overflow of activity from the right to the left hemisphere, or if the left hemisphere is particularly vulnerable to such interhemispheric activity, we should expect stutterers to have more difficulty than non-stutterers in performing two different motor activities with the two hands simultaneously. (A split-brain patient should have little difficulty doing such a task because without an intact corpus callosum, the hemispheres are not connected to one another at least at the cortical level). In several experiments I found greater difficulty experienced by the stutterers in performing bimanual coordination tasks requiring the performance of two tasks simultaneously.

As one example, participants were required to perform either the repetitive sequential finger tapping task (Webster, 1986a) or the sequence reproduction task (Webster, 1989a), as described earlier, using the right hand, and to perform **concurrently** a second task that required them to **turn a knob** back and forth with the left hand whenever a tone sounded. Not surprisingly, all participants, both stutterers and non-stutterers, showed an interference effect whereby the knob turning interfered with finger tapping. The critical finding for our purpose was that the participants who stuttered showed significantly **more interference** compared to the fluent control participants. In other words, in stutterers, left hand (right hemisphere) activity interfered more than in controls with concurrent right hand (left hemisphere) finger movements. Presumably this interference occurred through neurons comprising the corpus callosum that interconnects the two hemispheres.

In another experiment (Webster, 1988), we found a similar differential interference effect using a **bimanual handwriting task**. On each trial the participant was required to write, using both hands simultaneously, the first letter of four words that had just been read aloud. Writing was done on two upright surfaces (fashioned after the "critical angle board" of Van Riper, 1934) with a black cloth draped over the apparatus to block the participants' view of their hands. The participants who stuttered not only took longer than the non-stutterer controls to write the four letters, but they made more errors than the controls, particularly errors that were mirror reversals (*e.g.*, **b** instead of **d**) usually by the left hand). These results were consistent with the interference model. So, to expand our earlier generalization about brain organization in people who stutter,

> *the left hemisphere motor control mechanisms in stutterers*
> *are susceptible to interference from other neural activities,*
> *particularly those of the right hemisphere.*

The generalization does not specify whether the susceptibility is due to overactivity in the right hemisphere or to a "fragility" or "vulnerability" of the left hemisphere mechanisms, or both. But, first, which left hemisphere mechanisms are involved?

Reflection Note to the Reader

How might the differences between stutterers and non-stutterers on the sequence reproduction task play out in learning and performing a musical instrument like the piano or violin by musicians who stutter? In other contexts? What do the group differences on the bimanual handwriting task suggest one would find in other analogous contexts?

---

* * * * * * * *

The original sequence reproduction finger tapping study (Webster, 1986a) led me to suspect that a key area of the brain that is implicated in stuttering is the **supplementary motor area** (SMA). For those with some familiarity with neuroanatomy, the SMA is part of the frontal lobe and is located on the medial bank of the hemispheres just above the cingulate cortex and anterior to the hind limb region of the primary motor cortex (Tanji, 1994). First called the supplementary motor area by Penfield and Welch (1949), based on their clinical research involving electrical stimulation of exposed cerebral cortex of human patients, the area was the subject of much research attention in human and non-human subjects starting in the 1960s and 70s. A number of methodologies were used in that and subsequent research, including the analysis of regional cerebral blood flow, positron emission tomography, DC electrical potentials, single neuron recordings, electrical stimulation, and the neuropsychological analysis of behavioural effects of lesions in both humans and animals, together with basic research on neuroanatomy. Goldberg (1985), Tanji (1994), and Wise (1984) have reviewed the research literature in the area, and a number of consistent sets of findings emerged that pointed to SMA function in the normal organization of behavior. I mention only four that seem especially germane for this discussion on stuttering.

First, as evidenced in single cell recording studies of nonhuman primates (Mushiake, Inase, & Tanji, 1990; Tanji & Shima (1994) as well as in brain imaging studies of human subjects (Roland, 1984a,1984b), activity in the SMA is associated with the **planning of complex sequential movements of either the limbs or the speech musculature** (Ikeda, Luders,

Shibasaki, Collura, Burgess, Morris, & Hamano, 1995). The critical words here are "**planning**," "**complex**," and "**sequential**". The area does **not** seem to be critically involved in the execution of well-practiced or simple movements but shows evidence of increased activity when the person is simply thinking about carrying out an action or when the movement involves a number of components (Simonetta, Clanet, & Roscol, 1991; Wohlert, 1993). These findings are consistent with reports from human patients that electrical stimulation of the area results in a **feeling of intention to move** (Penfield & Welch, 1949), but the stimulation does not result in movement as such. Electrical stimulation also interferes with speech, specifically resulting in slowing, hesitation, and an inability to initiate speech sounds (Ojemann, 1983).

These observations parallel the difficulties reported for people who stutter with respect to speech initiation (Bloodstein, 1981), the performance of mirror-symmetric movements (Webster, 1988), and the organization and initiation of new nonspeech response sequences (Webster, 1986a) discussed earlier. The parallels lead directly to the hypothesis that the underlying neurological basis of stuttering is to be found, at least in part, in compromised SMA integrity. A similar conclusion was reached by Caruso, Abbs, and Gracco (1988) on the basis of their elegant analysis of the spatial and temporal aspects of lip and jaw movements in the fluent speech of people who stutter.

In 1964, Professor H.H. Kornhuber and his colleagues at university hospital Freiburg im Breisgau, reported finding a very small amplitude but consistent electrical potential that they called the "Bereitschaftspotential," German for "readiness potential." The potential was recorded through electrodes connected to the scalp, as used in recording the electroencephalogram (EEG), and it becomes evident through the use of signal averaging techniques. It was found to immediately precede the initiation of a voluntary movement, like a finger movement, by roughly one-half second. The early part of the potential was found to be generated by the SMA and the latter part, which immediately followed the start of the movement, was found to be generated by the primary motor cortex. The name of the electrophysiological potential was derived from the fact that the first part of it seemed to reflect the brain "getting ready" to make a voluntary movement rather than actually making the movement itself.

In the context of the interhemispheric interference I discussed earlier, the characteristics of the readiness potential suggest, provocatively, that the vulnerability of the left hemisphere SMA to interference from other brain activity may be through whatever SMA neuronal processes are reflected in the readiness potential.

The **second** point is that there are rich intra- and inter-hemispheric connections involving the SMA (Goldberg, 1985). In fact, most inter-hemispheric connections between the motor areas go through the SMA (Rouiller et al., 1994) and normally the two SMAs operate in a coordinated manner.

The **third** set of findings implicates the SMA as being crucial in bimanual coordination (Lang et al., 1990): In both patients and non-human primates, damage to the SMA interferes with the ability to coordinate hand movements and to do two different things with the hands at the same time (Brinkman, 1984).

The **fourth** set of findings provides evidence that the area is crucial for the planning of **self-initiated and internally guided movements** (and speech would involve such movements) rather than ones that are externally signaled and externally guided (Halsband et al., 1994; Passingham, 1989). Such guidance likely involves the use of kinesthesis, the awareness of the position and movement of the parts of the body by means of **proprioceptors** in the muscles and joints. In chapter 6, I will be discussing the research of David Forster, which bears on neural correlates of recovery from stuttering. However, one part of his research findings is particularly germane to this present question of kinesthesis and internally guided movement.

One of the motor control tasks that David Forster (1996) devised for his dissertation research was a computer-based version of Preilowski's (1972) **bimanual crank turning task**, similar in principle to an "Etch A Sketch®" child's toy. In the toy version, two knobs control the X-Y movements of a "cursor" which leaves a track on a screen as the knobs are turned. In Forster's study, instead of a pair of knobs there was a pair of balanced cranks mounted side by side on a metal chassis and interfaced with a computer and flat-screen monitor. Turning the cranks moved a computer cursor. One crank controlled the up/down movement and the other controlled the left/right movement, and the movement of the cursor left a trace of the cursor's path on the screen. The task for the participant was to turn the cranks at the correct relative speed in order to move the cursor so it stayed inside two parallel guidelines on the screen. When the track angle was 26.5 degrees, successful performance required the right hand to turn twice as quickly as the left; when the angle was 63.5 degrees, it required the left hand to turn twice as quickly as the right. This is a task that clearly involved hand coordination. Performance was determined basically by the time required to move the cursor to the top of the guidelines. The deviation of the cursor track from a straight line within the guidelines was the dependent variable of principal interest.

The key experimental manipulation relevant for this present discussion was that on half the trials, the visual display of the cursor was shut off part way up the track, and the task for the participant was to continue to turn the cranks at the same rates used at the beginning of the trial. Performance under this non-visually guided condition required reliance on proprioceptive or kinesthetic cues from muscles and joints.

The participants included i) adults who currently stutter, ii) adults who reported having stuttered as children but no longer did so (ex-stutterers), and iii) adults of similar age and backgrounds who reported never having stuttered. They were tested on the bimanual crank turning task as well as other experimental tasks I will return to in chapter 6. At this juncture, I will focus only on the performance adults who currently stutter and the control participants who had never stuttered. (This is the comparison made in the other studies described in this chapter). A key finding (Forster & Webster, 2001) was that the **non-visually guided** cursor traces for the group that stuttered were 40% less accurate than for the controls who did not. However, when **visual feedback** was available, the two groups were similar in accuracy. In other words, when the participants in both groups were able to see the cursor track and adjust their crank turning in response as needed to this feedback, performance was similar. When participants could not see the cursor track and had to guide their crank turning using proprioceptive or kinesthetic cues from the muscles, the stutterers made more errors and were slower than the fluent controls. This finding highlights the importance of proprioceptive or kinesthetic cues in under-standing the speech motor control mechanisms of people who stutter.

* * * * * * * *

If the left hemisphere SMA is vulnerable to interference from the right hemisphere, what is going on in the right hemisphere to produce the inter-ference, and to produce interference that varies across time and situations?

The possibility that is highly relevant for understanding stuttering comes from the substantial body of electrophysiological research (Ahern & Schwartz, 1985; Davidson, 1984; Davidson & Fox 1981; Fox & Davidson, 1988) suggesting that when **positive emotions** are experienced that moti-vate us to **approach** a situation, the **left** hemisphere becomes increasingly active. In contrast, and this is a critical part, when **negative emotions** like fear, apprehension, shame, or embarrassment are experienced, all emo-tions that motivate us to **withdraw** from a situation, the **right** hemisphere becomes increasingly active.

This leads to the idea of a feedback loop which, in principle, has the following elements:

- the fear and anxiety and apprehension related to stuttering are associated with right hemisphere activation,
- this activation in turn interferes with the left hemisphere SMA,
- the interference results in discoordination and stuttering, and
- the stuttering then reinforces the fear and apprehension of being in the speech situation.

In other words, I envisage a feedback system through which the neurol-ogy of stuttering and the psychology of stuttering intersect.

However, as I will go on to describe in chapter 6, the situation with right hemisphere activation is more complex than was assumed in our initial Interference Model. Before we move on to that discussion, it is important to end this chapter with an acknowledgement of the contribution of one particular organization to this research program.

Carleton University Science Technology Centre

Any research program involves people other than the principal investiga-tors. I have mentioned in various places some individuals by name, and

I have made reference to the Natural Sciences and Engineering Research Council which provided grant support for this research. But I want to briefly spotlight the Science Technology Centre at Carleton University that worked with me to design and fabricate much of the research equipment I used in my research on stuttering. This is a good example of invaluable research infrastructure found in universities but often out of view of the general public.

In the post-World War II years, when Carleton University was evolving into a comprehensive university with an emphasis on research and graduate programs in a full range of disciplines, its leadership had the foresight to develop and fund what was called the Science Technology Centre. It was a well-equipped machine-, electronics-, woodworking-, and metal-shop comprised at the time of more than 20 highly skilled technicians. The technicians in the Centre could design and build almost anything for research, and it charged Carleton researchers remarkably modest rates. I understood that the whole operation was held together financially through external contracts with major research and development initiatives, both in Canada and internationally. The Centre is still in operation today and, as it notes in its current website description, "our parts have been installed underground as part of CERN and sent into space with NASA!" But more importantly for me, the Centre is what made my research possible.

The two electronics technicians with whom I worked were Bill Ferguson and Mike Jutting. They had been working at the time to develop various electronic timers and counter modules, as well as generic control modules, that could be easily wired together for use in experimental psychology experiments like mine. In the year I was getting tooled up, they taught a short hands-on course for graduate students and faculty on the use of integrated logic circuit chips for controlling the modules. Taking this course proved valuable for me for at least three reasons.

First, it taught me what this technology could actually do, what its limitations are, and how it could be used to control psychology experiments.

Second, the course also taught me how to design and wire together simple circuits. This meant that I did not have to be totally dependent on the staff to make minor modifications or additions to the circuits when there were changes to the protocols.

The third, and particularly valuable part of this course, was that it taught me the language of the technology, and that in turn allowed me to discuss easily with Bill and Mike my equipment needs and the logic circuits that would be required. Both were superb in understanding the needs of this psychology professor and they were able to design and fabricate much of the equipment that was required in the studies described in these chapters.

I extend my deep gratitude to Bill and Mike, and to the Carleton leadership for this key infrastructure that supported (and still supports) faculty and student research.

CHAPTER 6

The Brain of the Person who Stutters: Hemisphere Activation

As my research studies continued with Joanne Hakkaku as my research assistant, it became apparent that things were more complicated with the right hemisphere than had been suggested by our earlier studies. My sense of this emerged from a study (Webster, 1987) designed to see if the origin of the interference effects we had found previously were specific to right hemisphere activity or might be more generalized and evident with other kinds of concurrent cognitive and motor processes.

The initial task I devised to test this question of **generalized** versus **specific** origins of interference used the **rapid letter-sequence transcription task**, a form of speech-shadowing (Treisman, 1965). This required the research participants to transcribe to paper rapidly presented letter sequences (such as N A S B O C R) of progressively longer length, from three to ten letters, and presented aurally at a rate faster than could be written simultaneously. Writing was done with the dominant right hand. Successful performance required concurrent monitoring and writing, and there was no reason to believe that these processes, which seemingly are more attentionally than motorically demanding, involve the interhemispheric processes that we encountered with the finger tapping and concurrent motor response tasks.

On a number of accuracy and time performance variables, the participants who stuttered performed more poorly than controls in their letter sequence transcriptions. In a subsequent study, I also found them to perform more poorly than controls if required to write the letters using recall immediately after the presentation of the sequences was complete (Webster 1990b). The results of the two studies paralleled those involving sequence reproduction performance and were consistent with the idea that stuttering is a phenomenon not restricted to disfluent speech production; it may reflect a more general difficulty with motor and cognitive organization. I started to think that part of the difficulty with organization might involve attentional processes related to hemisphere activation.

Chapter 5 discussed the distinction between hemisphere lateralization and hemisphere specialization. A substantial body of literature in neuropsychology (Bradshaw & Nettleton 1983; Bryden, 1982) supported a further distinction between hemisphere specialization and hemisphere activation.

On the one hand, the concept of **hemisphere specialization** refers to the underlying structural specializations of the hemispheres (e.g., speech and language versus spatial processing), as discussed in chapter 5.

On the other hand, the concept of **hemisphere activation** refers to the influence of the ascending reticular activating system (ARAS) on the forebrain. This is part of what is called the reticular formation situated diffusely in the midbrain and hindbrain regions and projecting through the thalamus to the cerebral cortex. The ARAS plays a key role in maintaining behavioural arousal and consciousness including alertness and attention. Its influence on the cerebral hemispheres is evident in patterns of electrophysiological activity (EEG) activity recorded from the two hemispheres and is manifest cognitively in the distribution of attentional resources favouring one side of the body or the other, or one side of space or the other (Bryden, 1982). Right hemisphere arousal would direct attention more to the left than right perceptual space, and left hemisphere arousal would direct attention more to the right than left perceptual space. The differential arousal or activation of the hemispheres could be either an **enduring and on-going bias** (i.e., one hemisphere is always more ready to attend and respond) or a **transient** activation bias dependent on the nature of the specific task being performed. I will return to this shortly; it may be both. In the meantime, the distinction and the evidence for it led to yet another generalization about brain organization in people who are fluent:

> *Through the brainstem ascending reticular activating system (ARAS), the two cerebral hemispheres can be differentially engaged or activated to reflect the attentional demands of the situation.*

Tied to this concept of hemisphere activation is the concept of **an inherent bias towards left hemisphere activation**, sometimes referred to as **utilization bias** (McGilchrist, 2010). This concept is derived from a number of lines of evidence, including those from the study of perceptual asymmetries in experimental neuropsychology using dichotic listening or visual perceptual half-field methodologies (Annett, 1978; Bryden, 1978; Cohen, 1982; Bryden & Mondor, 1991; Mondor & Bryden, 1992; McGilchrist, 2010). This evidence indicates that **right-handers** have a predisposition for the left hemisphere to be in a tonic state of greater readiness than the right hemisphere to process information and to respond (i.e., it is in a heightened state of attention to right perceptual space). I stress right-handers because **left-handers** (again, I am referring to people who do not stutter) do not appear to have this bias but are able to direct their attention equally readily to right and left perceptual space.

One nice demonstration of this concept was provided by Peters (1987) who developed a task that required participants to tap a telegraphic key twice with one hand for every single tap of another key by the other hand. Peters reported that right-handed non-stutterers performed this task better when it was the right hand that tapped twice (R2/L1 condition) rather than when it was the left hand that tapped twice (L2/R1 condition). Among left-handed non-stutterers, however, performance was similar under the two lead-hand tapping conditions. Drawing upon Annett's (1978) single gene model of handedness, which proposed that right-handers but not left-handers have this inherent directional bias, Peters argued that the differences he observed between right- and left-handers reflected the role of attention in the expression of handedness. More specifically, he argued that right-handers have an attentional bias to the right hand (left hemisphere) that facilitated performance in the R2/L1 condition. In contrast, left-handers are more flexible in focusing lateralized attention and can attend with equal facility with either the right or left hand leading. Underlying this right-side attention bias in right-handers is an on-going or tonic left hemisphere activation which is not found in left-handers; as a result, left-handers show greater lability of hemisphere activation.

This kind of evidence on hemisphere activation bias and handedness in fluent speakers leads to a further generalization about lateralization that will be particularly germane in a moment to the issue of stuttering:

> *An inherent bias towards the left hemisphere activation is found in right-handed fluent speakers: a more equal distribution of activation (and attention) is found in left-handed fluent speakers.*

So, which hemisphere activation pattern, if either, is demonstrated by people who stutter? The pattern shown in fluent right-handers, or the pattern shown by fluent left-handers? Something else? As emerges from the research studies I will describe, the pattern in stutterers (both left and right handed) is like that of fluent **left-handers** (and different from fluent right-handers).

When I repeated the Peters (1987) study with participants who stutter (Webster, 1990a), I found that both right- and left-handed stutterers performed like the left-handed non-stutterers (in other words, with similar performance under the two lead hand conditions). Following from Peters' interpretation of the lead-hand performance symmetry in left-handers, I interpreted the results with participants who stuttered as indicating that they (both right- and left-handers) **lack** a left hemisphere activation bias and have greater lability or flexibility of hemisphere activation. This lability might provide a hint as to why the right hemisphere can become overactive in stutterers under some circumstances.

Before I explore that hint, I need to describe one other experiment that had a different purpose and methodology but led to a similar conclusion about hemisphere activation in people who stutter.

The study (Forster & Webster, 1991) was designed to determine whether the dual task interference results described previously were specific to tasks that involved opposite hemispheres, as implied by the Interhemispheric Interference Model illustrated in figure 2, or whether interference would also be observed when any two tasks are performed concurrently, including when the two tasks are mediated primarily by one hemisphere. This is another way of asking the generalized versus specific interference question, similar to that asked by the rapid letter transcription task (Webster, 1987) previously described.

The paradigm was similar to that used in one of the dual task interference studies (Webster, 1986b) previously described. In that study, the research participants were asked to perform **finger tapping** with one hand while performing concurrently a **stimulus-contingent knob turning task** (i.e., "turn the knob back and forth each time a tone sounds"). In this present study, the participants were tested on a repetitive sequential finger tapping task with one hand (either right or left hand) while the concurrent task was modified to involve **pressing a foot pedal** in response to a tone onset using either the contralateral foot (inter-hemispheric pairing) or ipsilateral foot (intra-hemispheric pairing). This means that each participant was tested under four hand and foot conditions (RH-RF; RH-LF; LH-RF; LH-LF).

Two major findings emerged from the concurrent task analysis. First, both the stutterers and non-stutterers showed greater interference on finger tapping with the **intra**-hemispheric hand-foot pairing compared to the **inter**-hemispheric pairing (for example, right hand and right foot versus right hand and left foot). This was not a result that was expected, and it was intriguing because the foot pedal task, like the letter transcription task, was arguably more attentionally than motorically demanding. This perspective made finding the effect in both groups particularly interesting in the context of hemisphere activation and attention.

Further analysis of the data, focusing on a more detailed look at the different hand and foot combinations, provided some insight.

There was a difference between the two groups, stutterers and non-stutterers, in the impact of concurrent right vs. left foot responding on the finger tapping. The non-stuttering control participants showed more interference when they were using the **left** foot (controlled by the right hemisphere) compared to using the **right** foot (controlled by the left hemisphere) to respond, regardless of which hand was being used for finger tapping. We interpreted this finding for the non-stutterers in terms of the attentional demands that the foot-responding task placed on a system with an inherent left hemisphere attention bias. The use of the left foot, controlled by the right hemisphere, required a shift of attention from the activation-biased left hemisphere to the right hemisphere each time the signal sounded. When using the right foot, controlled by the left hemisphere, no such shift was required because of the continuing left hemisphere activation bias. By contrast, among the participants who stuttered and who, as discussed earlier, appear to lack a left hemisphere activation bias, the impact of the concurrent foot responding task on finger tapping performance was found to be the same for right and left foot responding. The lack of difference between the two feet with respect to interference is consistent with the idea that stutterers have a relatively labile system of hemisphere activation that can readily switch activation between the hemispheres.

The convergence of conclusions from the two very different studies provides a basis for some confidence that the hypothesized mechanisms warrant a generalization about brain organization in people who stutter, specifically that,

> People who stutter (right- or left-handed) do not demon-
> strate the left hemisphere activation bias found in right-
> handed fluent speakers but are similar to left-handed fluent
> speakers by showing a distribution of hemisphere activation
> (and attention) that is more equal, flexible, and labile.

Two comments on this generalization:

First, the overlap between the patterns of hemisphere activation in stutterers and in left-handed non-stutterers does raise the question about whether stutterers are more prone than non-stutterers to be left-handed. There is a long history to this question (Coren, 1992; Kushner, 2011), going back at least as far as Orton (1928) and Travis (1931) who claimed such an association. Subsequent research produced mixed and inconclusive results. In my laboratory (Webster & Poulos, 1987), we carried out an analysis of previously collected handedness data from our various clinical and research samples of stutterers. The analysis provided no support for an association between left-handedness and stuttering. Stutterers had neither a greater incidence of left-handedness than is usually reported for the general population, nor demonstrated less consistency and strength of hand preference compared to non-stutterers. That said, in my view this question is more complicated than it appears, and I keep an open mind about it. I also keep an open mind on a second and related question of whether the practice, not uncommon even a generation ago, of forcing a left-handed child to switch their writing hand can lead to stuttering onset. There is a long history with mixed results on this second question as well (Coren, 1992; Kushner, 2011). The Two-Factor Interference Model of Stuttering to be discussed shortly suggests that theoretically there may well be **some conditions** under which a forced dominant hand change could result in stuttering onset. But that is a question for another day when there are more systematic research data available bearing directly on the matter.

Second, this quality among stutterers to have flexible hemisphere activation or attention is reflected in the attenuated ear and visual-field asymmetries in stutterers compared to non-stutterers on dichotic listening tasks (e.g., Blood, 1985; Brady & Berson, 1975; Curry & Gregory, 1969; Rosenfield & Goodglass, 1980) and tachistoscopic visual half-field recognition tasks (e.g., Johannsen & Victor, 1986; Moore, 1976), respectively. This attention-based interpretation of reduced perceptual asymmetries has come to be favoured (e.g., Peters, 1987) over the earlier 1970s interpretation of the asymmetries reflecting representation of speech processes as discussed early in chapter 5. Personally, I suspect that perceptual asymmetries actually reflect the interplay of both hemisphere specialization and hemisphere activation processes, with the outcome dependent on the specific task demands in the research studies.

Reflection Note to the Reader

The reader may find it interesting to speculate on what positive or negative qualities other than those related to speech might be associated with or facilitated by the hemisphere activation lability or flexibility shared by people who stutter and by fluent *left*-handers. Might there be advantages to having the two hemispheres able to communicate easily with one another? Might there be disadvantages?

Figure 3 represents conceptually where all this research has led me (Webster, 2004). The model is similar to the Interhemispheric Interference Model illustrated in figure 2, but it has a refinement: it incorporates the idea of a labile pattern of hemisphere activation. The two factors referred to in the name of this model are:

- the **speech motor control system**, including its susceptibility to interference from right hemisphere neural activities, as in figure 2; and
- the **hemisphere activation** differences between stutterers and non-stutterers, more specifically the lack, in people who stutter, of the left hemisphere activation bias found in right-handed (but not left-handed) fluent speakers.

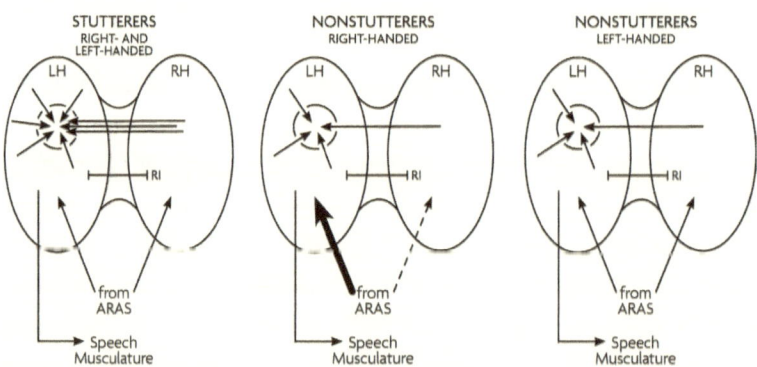

Figure 3. Two-factor Interference Model of Stuttering. LEFT DIAGRAM: Right- and left-handed stutterers; MIDDLE DIAGRAM: Right-handed non-stutterers; RIGHT DIAGRAM: Left-handed non-stutterers. (LH=left hemisphere; RH=right hemisphere; RI=reciprocal inhibition; ARAS=ascending reticular activating system)

In this model:

- The supplementary motor area (SMA) of the left hemisphere is represented by the small circle.
- The vulnerability of the SMA to interference from other brain activity is represented by the "pores" in each small circle, as well as by the varying number and origin of interference arrows.
- Although some interference may be of intra-hemisphere origin (the shorter arrows within the hemisphere), interference of inter-hemispheric origin and mediated through the corpus callosum (the longer arrows from one hemisphere to the other) is of particular significance for understanding variation in stuttering severity.
- Hemisphere activation is represented by the arrows from the ARAS to each hemisphere.
    - A broad arrow projecting to the left hemisphere combined with a narrow and dashed arrow projecting to the right hemisphere is used to indicate the left hemisphere activation bias of right-handed fluent speakers.
    - To indicate the labile and non-biased hemisphere activation system found both in left-handed non-stutterers and in right- and left-handed stutterers, equally narrow arrows are shown projecting to the right and left hemispheres.
- RI refers to reciprocal inhibition between the hemispheres, a process whereby increased activation in one hemisphere leads to increased inhibition and hence decreased activation of the other (Kinsbourne, 1977; McGilchrist, 2010). This process has the effect of magnifying the difference between the hemispheres in information processing.

* * * * * * * *

Before getting into what this model may mean for understanding the dynamics of stuttering and its implications for the management of speech by people who stutter, I will take a slight detour to discuss how the model provided a conceptual platform for a study on understanding neural mechanisms associated with recovery from childhood stuttering. The study, part of David Forster's doctoral research (Forster, 1996; Forster & Webster, 2001), was introduced in chapter 5 in the context of kinesthesis.

It compared the performance of 1) adults who currently stutter (**persistent stutterers**), 2) adults who reported having stuttered as children but no longer did so (**ex-stutterers**), and 3) adults of similar age and backgrounds who reported never having stuttered (**control participants**) on two sets of tasks. One set focused on the speech-motor control factor and other set focused on the hemisphere activation factor.

By way of background, it is estimated that as many as 80 percent of young children who stutter recover spontaneously without formal treatment (Andrews et al., 1983; Andrews & Harris, 1964). The remaining children persist in their stuttering through adulthood. Risk factors for persistent stuttering include late onset of speech, being male, disfluencies persisting for more than twelve to eighteen months, and a family history of stuttering. (My own profile contains all these risk factors). Factors associated with recovery from stuttering include typical speech and language skills, decreasing disfluencies with time, being female, and no family history of stuttering. If the Two-Factor Interference Model we have been exploring here has value, it should have something to contribute to our understanding of mechanisms of recovery from stuttering.

The first set of experimental tasks used by Forster (1996), intended to reflect the functioning of the SMA, included the **sequence reproduction finger tapping task** and **bimanual crank turning task**, both of which were described earlier.

The second set of experimental tasks was intended to tap into the hypothesized anomaly in hemisphere activation also described earlier. The tasks were two tachistoscopic divided visual field tasks: a verbally based **lexical decision task** and a spatially based **dot enumeration task**.

The procedures for the lexical decision task were based on those described by Mondor and Bryden (1992). The stimuli consisted of 40 three-letter **words** and 40 pronounceable three-letter **non-words**, and they were presented briefly on a white background on a computer monitor. The task was to identify as quickly and as accurately as possible whether each stimulus was a word or a non-word by pressing one button or another. Participants were tested under both a **cued condition**, wherein a pre-cue (blue dot) was presented 67 msec before the target stimulus in the visual field into which the target stimulus would appear, and a **non-cued**

condition wherein the blue dot and target stimulus were presented simultaneously. After 32 practice trials, each of the 80 different test stimuli was presented once to each visual field for a total of 160 trials. Previous research had indicated that most right-handed adults perform better when the word/non-word verbal material is presented to the right visual field (which projects to the left hemisphere).

The dot enumeration task used the same equipment and similar procedures as described for the lexical decision task. In this case, the stimuli consisted of 160 different arrangements of from **three to six dots** (diameter=2 mm) presented inside a 2 cm x 2 cm line frame that served as the pre-cue. The task of the participants was to indicate, using response keys, whether there had been an **even number** or **odd number** of dots presented. Previous research has indicated that most right-handed adults perform better on this non-verbal task when the material is presented to the left visual field (which projects to the right hemisphere).

On the **two motor control tasks** thought to be sensitive to SMA function, the recovered or **ex-stutterers** performed the same as **non-stutterers**, and both of these now-fluent groups performed better than the participants who were **persistent stutterers.**

On **the lexical decision task**, one of the two tests thought to be sensitive to hemisphere activation, the control participants who had never stuttered showed the usual and expected right visual field advantage (reflecting the left hemisphere activation bias). However, the other two groups, comprised of the participants who **stuttered** and the participants who had once stuttered (the **ex-stutterers**), were similar to one another in showing no asymmetry, (i.e., **no hemisphere activation bias**). The data for the **dot enumeration task**, although based on the same measures and analyses used for the lexical decision task, were difficult to interpret because "overall performance on this task (particularly in the non-cued condition) was sufficiently poor as to make the reliability of the results questionable and the interpretation of the asymmetries problematic" (Forster & Webster, 2001, p. 139).

In summary, people who once stuttered as children but who no longer did so as adults (the ex-stutterers) showed evidence of now normal left hemisphere speech motor mechanisms, but they shared with persistent stutterers the lack of a left hemisphere activation bias.

Forster and Webster (2001) concluded that, taken together and being mindful of the weak results from the dot enumeration task, "the results from the four experimental tasks support the general hypothesis that an anomaly in interhemispheric relations and a deficit in the mechanisms for speech-motor control are each a necessary but not sufficient condition for stuttering, and that recovery from childhood stuttering reflects a maturation of the mechanisms of speech-motor control" (p. 142). Whatever maturation may have occurred with the speech motor mechanisms did not occur with the hemisphere activation mechanisms.

* * * * * * *

As described earlier, the Two-Factor Interference Model of stuttering illustrated in figure 3 includes a second factor not included in figure 2, a lack of the left hemisphere activation bias normally found in non-stutterers. The implication of this lack of bias is that it may contribute to the overactivation of the right hemisphere and hence may have an impact on speech.

The idea of right hemisphere overactivation in stutterers is not new and has attracted considerable interest over the years (Boberg et al., 1983; Moore, 1993; Moore & Haynes, 1980; Rastatter & Dell, 1987). What is perhaps original is what emerges from the **combination** of four ideas:

- right hemisphere overactivation contributes to stuttering by being a source of interference with left hemisphere processes, as discussed in chapter 5.
- although right hemisphere overactivation has been suggested by some to reflect ineffective attempts to process linguistic information by the right hemisphere (Moore, 1993; Rastatter & Dell, 1987), in my view a more compelling explanation was the one discussed in chapter 5: the association of positive (approach) and negative (avoidance, withdrawal) emotions and behaviour with left and right hemisphere activation, respectively (Ahern & Schwartz, 1985; Davidson, 1984; Davidson & Fox 1981; Fox & Davidson, 1988).
- reciprocal inhibition (Kinsbourne, 1977; McGilchrist, 2010), the process whereby increased activation of an area of one hemisphere

leads to the inhibition of the corresponding area of the opposite hemisphere, serves to amplify the differences in activation between the left and right hemispheres.

- in the absence of a left hemisphere activation bias in stutterers, there will be less tonic inhibition of the right hemisphere, making the right hemisphere predisposed to become more active than it would otherwise have been or than it is in people who do not stutter.

These ideas can be incorporated into the feedback loop discussed in chapter 5 so that in people who stutter:

- the right hemisphere has a predisposition to be active due to the lack of tonic inhibition from the left hemisphere;
- the right hemisphere is activated by the fear or anxiety or apprehension (negative withdrawal emotions) associated with speaking;
- right hemisphere activation means more inhibition of the left hemisphere SMA and more interference on left hemisphere SMA function;
- the stuttering reinforces the fear and apprehension of being in the speech situation, which further increases right hemisphere activation;
- the active generation or experience of positive (or approach) emotions or an increased focus on those speech motor movements that facilitate fluency will increase left hemisphere activation, and that will mean reduced right hemisphere activity due to reciprocal inhibition from the left hemisphere.

In its simplest form, as I will elaborate in chapter 9, the Two-Factor Interference Model suggests that the speech of people who stutter, *particularly those who have participated in a stuttering treatment program (like the Precision Fluency Shaping Program (PFSP), to be returned to in chapter 7) and have acquired speech motor skills that support fluent speech,* can be managed through a combination of

- focusing attention and activity in the left hemisphere SMA during speech production processing by deliberate use of fluency skills, and by amplifying kinesthetic feedback to the SMA from the oral musculature;

- reducing potential interference on the left hemisphere SMA from right hemisphere activation;
- preventing the right hemisphere from becoming overactivated.

Let me look at each of these in turn from the perspective of my personal experience.

With respect to the **first** point, I have often felt that when I used my fluency skills (as imperfect as they are) and really **felt** the movements through using slow and deliberate speech, my focus on and attention to those movements resulted in a feeling of control, as well as actual control, perhaps reflecting left hemisphere activation focused on the speech motor system. It seemed to me that a key part of the process of facilitating my fluency was to maximize kinesthetic feedback from the muscles and joints by actively **feeling** the speech motor movements as they were being made. As will be discussed in chapter 7, this is a key principle in the PFSP. David Forster's bimanual crank turning research discussed in chapter 5, suggested that the motor system of stutterers either does not have the same access to kinesthetic cues or does not have the same capacity to process kinesthetic cues to guide movements as does the motor system of fluent speakers. By trying to feel the muscle movements, kinesthetic cues are enhanced for the speech motor control system doing its work through the SMA to support movements for fluent speech.

Reflection Note to the Reader

A former colleague told me how, since childhood, he had always stuttered until he was in his mid-30s. He then had found inadvertently that when he intentionally adopted a slower, slightly exaggerated, and more deliberate speech style, his stuttering improved. This change in speaking style would have enhanced the kinesthetic feedback from the oral musculature.

When, in stutterers, speaking quality is purposively changed (e.g., speaking with a deeper or higher voice; speaking slower, faster; adopting a foreign accent), it is not unusual for fluency to improve, **but not for long**. It is largely a transient effect. What made my colleague's situation unusual was its unintentionality and the apparently persisting nature of the change. Over time, his new deliberate

---

style of speaking became increasingly habitual and automatic. He was comfortable with the style, and he claimed that his stuttering was behind him. When I knew him, no one ever suspected that he was a person who had stuttered. I had to take his word for it.

This brings me to the **second** point, the vulnerability of the left hemisphere SMA to interference from other brain activities.

The research literature discussed in the previous chapter suggested there are rich interhemispheric connections between the hemispheres through the corpus callosum making the left hemisphere SMA particularly susceptible to interference from right hemisphere activation. That interference starts when I come into a speaking situation with fears and apprehensions and that sense of impending loss of control, and it reflects (or creates) an elevated state of right hemisphere activation. The **absence** in me and other people who stutter of a left hemisphere activation bias may also mean that our right hemispheres tend to be prone to ready activation. I still feel at times that I live in the world of speech with a right hemisphere that is straining to get out of its cage and looking to bite my SMA, so to speak.

Reflection Note to the Reader

The Two-Factor Interference Model suggests that people who stutter who lack a left hemisphere activation bias generate less inhibition of the right hemisphere than non-stutterers. Could the resulting elevated levels of right hemisphere activity make people who stutter more susceptible than non-stutterers to experiencing negative emotions? Or is the experience of negative emotions amplified or more intense? Are people who stutter more emotionally labile than non-stutterers? Is the sense of an impending loss of control tied into elevated levels of right hemisphere activity?

On the **third** point, if right hemisphere overactivity is the problem, how can it be reduced? One way, as I will come back to in chapters 7 and 9, is to voluntarily bring under control negative emotions like fear and anxiety and apprehension as well as other factors that motivate us to withdraw from a situation, and to replace those emotions with positive ones that motivate us to enter the situation. When we control these kinds of emotions, I would like to think that we are voluntarily **reducing** activation of the right hemisphere and **enhancing** activation of the left. Enhancing activation of the left hemisphere can also be augmented, as noted above, by focusing attention on the motoric aspects of speech. Through reciprocal inhibition, that **increased** left hemisphere activity will further **decrease** right hemisphere activity and hence reduce interhemispheric interference. I recognize that the application of the theory, despite its apparent simplicity, is far easier said than done.

What may all this mean for the person who wants to become more fluent? How can one use all this theorizing? Briefly, and again anticipating chapters 7 and 9, I have often used **mental imaging** combined with the use of **more-effective self-talk** that we will discuss in chapter 7. If I am having difficulty starting to speak, or if I experience that sense of impending loss of control (as I often do), I consciously remind myself that my cerebral hemispheres just need to be adjusted. I conjure up a mental image of the two hemispheres interacting with one another and, using the kinds of more-effective self-talk to be described in chapter 7, I remind myself of the motor and emotional fluency skills over which I have some control. As I start to use those fluency skills, I imagine my left hemisphere increasing in size and my right hemisphere shrinking. This imaging approach of the feedback system doesn't always work, but it does provide a distraction from anxiety about my speech, and at the very least, I feel I have some control over the situation by exerting some control over my thoughts, emotions, and speech movements.

Brain Imaging Research

Up until this point, much of the cited research which led to the Two-Factor Interference Model has come from the world of experimental neuropsychology. How does more recent research on stuttering using regional cerebral blood flow (rCBF) neuroimaging methods like PET and fMRI scans fit with the Two-Factor Interference Model?

The mid- to late-1990s saw the first appearance of results of several neuroimaging studies of people who stutter. According to Ingham (2004), by 2002 five imaging studies had been published (Braun et al., 1997; De Nil et al., 2000; Fox et al., 1996; Ingham et al., 2000; Wu et al., 1995), each of which was designed to identify brain regions that are functionally related to stuttering. The particular imaging method used in these studies was either $H_2^{15}O$ positron emission tomography (PET scans) or functional magnetic resonance imaging (fMRI) to assess regional cerebral blood flow (rCBF). The assumption underlying the analysis was that changes in regional cerebral blood flow, or differences between groups in blood flow patterns, reflect the increased or decreased metabolic needs (for oxygen or glucose) of activated or inhibited neurons, respectively. Using a "subtraction technique," the images obtained during stuttered speech can be compared with those obtained from the same participants during, for example, induced (through choral reading) stutter-free speech (Braun et al., 1997; Fox et al., 1996) or from those obtained during speech of fluent control participants (De Nil et al., 2000). More robust analyses often take advantage of the variability of stuttering severity among participants and include an analysis of the correlations between severity of stuttering or stuttering symptoms and the amount of activation or deactivation in individual areas (Ingham, 2004).

Each of these studies has identified regions of the brain associated with stuttering in one form or another. Some areas of the brain showed activation and others showed de-activation. However, according to Ingham (2004), the consistency of results is poor across studies. After a detailed analysis of the findings of the five studies at the time, as well as an analysis restricted to the three $H_2^{15}O$ PET studies, he concluded that, "With the possible exception of unusual right hemisphere activations in the premotor area and deactivations in the auditory area, it appears that the differences among PET study findings grossly outweigh their 'similarities' (pp. 36-37)." This paucity of agreement undoubtedly reflects variations among studies in the details of the rCBF and speech task methodologies. It may also reflect the fact that regional brain activation results will include some speech and language processes that are associated with the **initiation** of speech, others which are the immediate **cause** of stuttering in the moment, others that relate to **language** rather than speech mechanics, others that relate to **emotional concomitants** of anticipating speech and stuttering, others which are **consequences** of speech, and probably a host of other considerations. How this plays out in an individual study will of course reflect the specific details of the methodology.

Even if the results of the analysis of rCBF images were to identify consistent stuttering-related regions of the brain, it is still not clear what one would do with the list to make it useful at this time. The list may tell you **what** is activated or deactivated in some specific speech context but little about **why** or **when**. However, neuroimaging technologies are powerful and ever evolving. And new technologies, like transcranial magnetic stimulation, are being developed and used in speech-related brain research (Ingham et al., 2018; Whillier et al., 2018). The enthusiastic optimism of a quarter century ago about imaging technologies answering our brain mechanism questions was perhaps premature, but I am cautiously optimistic that at some point the technology (perhaps incorporating the use of artificial intelligence) will catch up with the complexity of the neural circuits of interest to those of us who stutter. In the meantime, we may have to be content with more modest but hopefully still useful theories like the Two-Factor Interference Model.

Let me end this section by reminding you of the British statistician, George Box (1976), who I quoted in the Preface. He wrote, "All models are wrong, but some models are useful." The Two-Factor Interference Model I have been presenting here is without doubt incomplete and, in at least that sense, is wrong. For example, the model does not take account of the likely role of the basal ganglia/thalamocortical motor circuits in stuttering (Alm, 2004). Nonetheless, I have found the model as developed so far has been useful for my understanding and management of my own speech in most contexts, as was the earlier version of the model (the Interhemispheric Interference Model in figure 2) useful for the people who stutter with whom I worked years ago. I use the model to imagine what is going on in my brain as I experience that sense of impending loss of control or an actual loss of speech control. I use it to remind me of what I need to do to reduce right hemisphere activation. And I use it to remind me of what I need to do to try to enhance left hemisphere activation to support fluent speech. Much more on this in Part III.

CHAPTER 7

Lessons from Stuttering Treatment

Much of my understanding about stuttering and its treatment in adults reflects my reading of the clinical and neuroscientific literature, my professional collaboration with speech-language pathologists, my laboratory research, and of course my personal lifelong struggles and successes as a person who stutters. However, most importantly, my knowledge about adult stuttering is based on the opportunities I have had to interact with dozens of persons who stutter. They are the focus of attention in this chapter. I am grateful for the circumstances that led me to meet them and learn from them.

As my research plans began to fall into place, I realized that finding people who stutter to participate in my research experiments could be a challenge. Small newspaper advertisements and offering to pay participants can be effective recruitment techniques but, to put it rather coarsely, I was looking for a steady supply of participants. A colleague of mine, who was connected to what is now called the Ottawa Hospital Rehabilitation Centre, told me about an adult stuttering treatment program at the Centre and gave me the contact information for the two speech-language pathologists (SLPs) who ran that program. So, I eventually mustered up the courage to phone to ask if I might meet with them to discuss my developing a research program and whether they might be of assistance in recruiting participants. One SLP was Ms. Anne Godden, who was about to leave Ottawa to take a new position in speech-language pathology at Dalhousie University and the Nova Scotia Hearing and Speech Clinic (now known as Hearing and Speech Nova Scotia); the other was Ms. Marie Poulos who was replacing Anne. They agreed to meet me at the Centre.

I led off the conversation by describing my experiences with diet and stuttering that I have discussed earlier. I explained that this experience had motivated me to learn more about the biology of stuttering, and that I was interested in ultimately studying carbohydrate metabolism and its potential impact on speech. I focused the conversation, however, on how I planned to start my research program with a study designed to examine the Orton and Travis model. They were still interested.

I went on to explain that I would be approaching this research question using an analysis of finger tapping performance. As I tried to explain the rationale for this approach, it was clear that they were both becoming skeptical of this academic professor with peculiar ideas. I'm not sure whether the skepticism was about the possible diet connection or about the use of finger movements to study speech, or both, but some years later they both assured me that they had not actually been rolling their eyes. Nonetheless they were gracious in their response to my request for assistance in recruiting research participants. By coincidence, a new group of four or five adult clients who stuttered had just been formed and would be starting a three-week intensive treatment program the following week. I was assured I was welcome to meet with the group for a few minutes to explain what I wanted to do and why. The brief presentation to the clients went well and, if I recall correctly, all the clients were enthusiastic about participating.

(Parenthetically, who would have known that ten years later, after Anne had returned from Nova Scotia to Western University and I had left Carleton University and moved to Brock University in Niagara, our paths would cross again, some months after which we would be married? The world truly can be full of surprises).

After the group meeting on that following week, I met with Marie, who discussed with me in more detail the nature of the stuttering treatment program being offered at the Centre. She said I would be welcome to come to observe the group in future sessions if that would be of interest to me. It was. As I quickly learned, the program being followed at the Rehabilitation Centre had been developed by an American psychologist, Dr. R.L. Webster (1980), and was well known at the time. This was the *Precision Fluency Shaping Program* (PFSP) that was intended to be offered in an intensive group-based format. A small group of adults or adolescents who stutter would spend every weekday for three weeks learning and practicing making speech sounds using carefully controlled muscle movement patterns. Practicing was done both individually and in a group setting, and while much of the practice was done in the clinic, considerable emphasis was placed on using the newly acquired speech skills in the outside environment including at home. The goal of PSFP therapy was to correct the speech mechanics by replacing movements that lead to stuttering with movements that lead to fluency.

As Webster and Stoeckel (1984) explained in their client manual, the fundamental principle was that,

> ...*when the stutterer violates what are defined here as rules of speech mechanics, he will stutter. Conversely, when the stutterer remains within the physical boundaries defined by these rules, he will not stutter. The term speech mechanics is used to designate specific movement details involved in the act of talking. Certain movement details are characteristic of stuttered speech while other movement details are characteristic of fluent speech. The emphasis in this program is placed upon carefully changing the speech muscle movements of the person who stutters (p. 1).*

As is clear from this quotation, the focus of the PFSP (and many other stuttering treatment programs) was on modifying habitual muscle movements and acquiring new speech fluency skills. Acquiring any new movement pattern (think of sports, dance, playing piano or violin) requires **doing** and **practicing**, and then performing the new skill in progressively more challenging situations. **Thinking** and **talking** about stuttering is **not** what this is about; it's all about **doing** things regularly and consistently.

In the vocabulary of the PFSP, "details of speech muscle movement patterns, designated as targets, [are what] produce fluent speech sounds" (p. 8). These "targets," or speech fluency skills, relate to stretching sounds in a controlled way, breathing fully and coordinating the breath with the sound onset, using "gentle onsets" with different kinds of consonants and vowels, and linking sounds together smoothly. After years of using other movements, these new movement patterns can be difficult to learn and apply consistently. Webster and Stoeckel (1984) emphasized that "...therapy focusses on speech muscle movements" and that means that "attention should be directed primarily toward **feeling** your muscle movements and only secondarily to the sounds themselves" (p. 5).

Interestingly, in his book, *Principles of Psychology*, published in 1890, William James, a leading philosopher and psychologist in the early nineteenth century, argued that for one to perform some movement voluntarily, one must have a memory trace or an image or a sense in one's mind of what that movement feels like, in other words, the sensory consequences of contracting that muscle. Think of wiggling your ears. One of the reasons it is hard for most of us to do that is that we don't have a sense of what it feels like for our ear muscles to contract; that is because our ear muscles have not contracted before. The ears may have been passively moved (which does not involve a muscle contraction), but that does not provide the nervous system with sensory information about the desired outcome, the muscle contraction itself. Research early in the twentieth century (Bair, 1901, cited by Kimble & Perlmuter, 1970) showed that the application of mild electric shock delivered through small wire electrodes inserted into the external ear muscles (yes, the wires and the electrical current must have hurt) caused the ear muscle to contract, moving the ear. That movement activated muscle spindle receptors which produced a sensation of what the contracted muscle actually feels like. The results did not fully support the James' theory in that experiencing the sensation was not sufficient to immediately support voluntary ear movements. However, compared to participants who did not have the electrical stimulation, the treatment did facilitate subsequent trial and error learning using a mirror and facial gestures. The verbal responses of the participants indicated that the reaction to the electrical simulation gave them some idea or general guidance about what they were trying to do. As Kimble and Perlmuter (1970) noted, the research also indicated the importance of "focusing attention exclusively on the desired response, while at the same time ignoring others" (p. 375). This is in line with the emphasis in the PFSP on **feeling** movements. Deliberate oral movements, especially ones slightly exaggerated, help reinforce for the brain what the movements feel like. That feeling then, in turn, facilitates producing the movements voluntarily.

As was quite clear from their manual, Webster and Stoeckel (1984) believed that there is no place in treatment for a consideration of emotions or learning or other possible causes of or contributors to stuttering: "Only one basic idea is advanced here about the nature of stuttering: distorted speech muscle movements can be changed through the application of laboratory derived principles of learning" (p. 2).

The PFSP is still offered by speech-language pathologists, and other SLPs have developed their own approaches to treatment. For example, one program that has been offered for many years is the *Comprehensive Stuttering Program* (CSP) developed by Boberg and Kully (1985) at the Institute for Stuttering Treatment and Research (ISTAR) at the University of Alberta. It is not my intention to critique the PFSP or any other treatment program, or to provide much detail on the nature of PFSP targets or fluency skills, or to explain what is involved in learning these new speech movements. That is the domain of the speech-language pathologist working with a client. My describing muscle movements and a fluency shaping regimen would be no more helpful to a person who stutters and who strives for fluency than my describing in words how to play a passage from a piano sonata to a person who aspires to play the piano. From what we know from chapters 5 and 6 about the involvement of the left hemisphere SMA in stuttering, we can have some confidence that effective stuttering therapy needs to focus, as a minimum, on changing the mechanics of speech production in one way or another, as most present-day stuttering treatment programs do. That said, I would suggest that programs that place disproportionate emphasis on managing the emotional aspects of stuttering be viewed cautiously in light of the preponderance of neuroscientific research attesting to the organic origins of stuttering.

Shortly after my meetings with the first group, Marie raised with me whether I might meet with other groups two or three times during their three-week programs. I had learned a lot from that first group and enjoyed interacting with the participants. They apparently felt the same towards me and what we had done. I was keen to continue with other groups. I thought I could discuss my research (and current research of others) and encourage the clients to sign up as participants. I could also discuss more generally with the group the role of biological factors in stuttering (genetics, neurotransmitters, brain imaging) that Marie thought were important for the clients to know about, but which she did not feel entirely comfortable discussing herself. She also hoped that I would feel free to bring into the discussion with the groups my own experiences as a person who stutters. These meetings provided an opportunity for the clients to practice the fluency skills they were acquiring with a new person in the room. They also provided me with a wonderful window into the world of people who stutter that could help inform my research. Although I have stuttered my whole life, I had seldom met others who stuttered (we are all quite good at fading into the woodwork in social situations), and I had never had personal discussions of the sort I had with those first groups of clients.

Marie went on to tell me that, in her experience, clients had good immediate outcomes of therapy, but many clients faced challenges when trying to practice or transfer their new speech skills outside the clinic. In that context, some clients can become self-conscious, get overwhelmed, and be distracted by their long-held anxiety about speaking. As I met with a number of groups over the next many months, certain recurring themes ran through the discussions on this general topic of skill transfer. For example, clients felt:

- anxiety that, when using newly acquired fluency skills, the speech would sound slow and feel unnatural. In fact, during and after therapy when fluency skills are being used (hopefully consistently), the speech is usually slower than it had been, it is more controlled and deliberate, and it has fewer abrupt onsets, but the speech is fluent. One concern of the clients seemed to be how friends, family, and co-workers might interpret this change in speaking style.

- the impact of noticing tension through the body or having a sufficiently relaxed speech musculature, which in turn would distract from attending to fluency skills.
- a continued sense of an impending loss of control despite having new fluency skills, resulting in a continued tendency to avoid situations in which to practice skills.
- upset and frustration when things did not go as planned in using particular fluency skills in particular situations.
- social anxiety related to interacting with other people. Part of this reflected a lack of experience with the usual social scripts, for example, not knowing or not having practiced the "script" for making an introduction.

Much of the problem the clients experienced both with their stuttering and with using fluency skills seemed to boil down to self-talk. A colleague gave me a useful example of the self-talk he sometimes uses when making a presentation at a conference. If a member of the audience stands up and leaves the room while my colleague is speaking, rather than saying to himself something self-critical like, "My talk must be boring," my colleague says to himself, "That poor person is going to miss the rest of my great presentation." What we say to ourselves about events, our self-talk has an impact on our interpretation of and our emotional reactions to events.

I saw parallels between what I had been discussing with the clients and how sport psychology facilitates the performance of athletes in analogous situations. It is not unusual for athletes who have well-developed skills to encounter difficulty in using their skills optimally in competition. Negative self-talk can be the culprit: the person telling themselves that they can't win, or that they are going to be distracted when they perform, or they tense up, or they conjure up memories of past competitions in which they felt they had failed (even though they did well, but not quite well enough to win the event). Sport psychologists work with athletes to optimize their performance by reducing cognitive and emotional interference on their performance and maximizing facilitating factors. Sport psychologists don't train the athlete; they work with the athlete to minimize distractors and to maximize focus and performance. And for a person in stuttering therapy, practicing new fluency skills at home or in the community is very much comparable to conditions in sports of high stress and "competition."

I suggested to Marie that her clients may have needed help to ferret out what specifically was interfering with their use of fluency skills in their speaking, how these interfering factors could be counteracted, and what could be done to facilitate performance. As I attended various professional conferences at the time, I became aware that these issues of "transfer and maintenance of fluency," as they are called, were not unique to the Rehabilitation Centre's program but were ubiquitous in stuttering therapy. Perhaps, I suggested, I could introduce the clients in my group sessions to what sport psychologists do with athletes.

As various groups progressed through the program during the following year or two, a time period that paralleled progress in my laboratory research, I developed what amounted to a curriculum for each session. Through our open and free-wheeling group discussions, I came to understand the various reasons why the clients had difficulty transferring their skills from the clinic to the community. I also heard their individual stories as people who stuttered. I could easily relate to and respond with empathy to their speech-related fears, anxieties, and difficult experiences, many of which were similar to my own. I also came to see how positive and liberating the newly found fluency was for most. I continued to consider how I might adapt performance-enhancing strategies from the world of sports to performance enhancement in the world of stuttering therapy. I also became quite familiar with the nature of the fluency skills on which the clients were working during the three weeks of the program. I was careful, however, not to go beyond occasionally reminding the clients to use their fluency skills while participating in our group discussions. I say, "occasionally" because the conversations we had together were sometimes challenging, and the clients and I found that focusing on the **how** of speech (using fluency skills like, for example, controlled breathing and gentle onsets) could interfere with the more immediate issue of the moment, the **what** and **why** of the experience being discussed.

The notes and handouts for the group discussions slowly expanded, ideas were fleshed out, worksheets were refined, and eventually we thought we had the makings of a manual that could be published and used in this and other stuttering treatment programs. It was published in 1989 as *Facilitating Fluency: Transfer Strategies for Adult Stuttering Treatment Programs* (Webster & Poulos, 1989).[1] Figure 4, reprinted from the manual, shows schematically how we came to conceptualize the problems the clients faced. **One key concept** was that it is primarily through the use of fluency skills that fluency and communication are enhanced. One can tell oneself repeatedly "I'm not going to stutter," or "I can do this," or "I'll just introduce myself—no problem today, even though I stuttered badly on my name yesterday," but without the skills (motor or cognitive), little will change. The **second key concept** is that there are some factors that interfere with the use of fluency skills (which result in stuttering and poor communication), and there are other factors that can facilitate the use the skills (and hence facilitate fluency and communication).

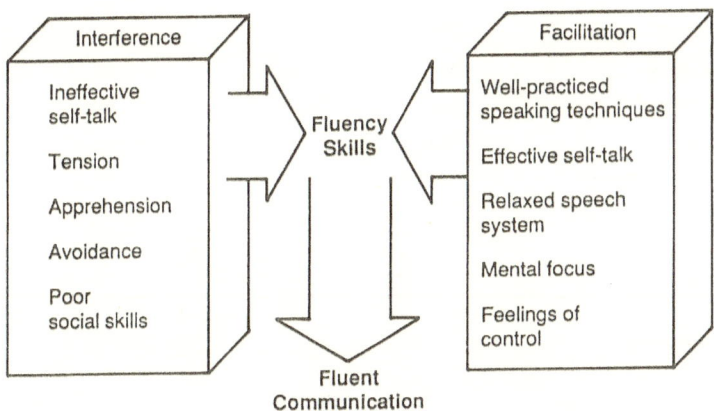

Figure 4. A representation of factors that may facilitate and factors that may interfere with the successful use of fluency skills in everyday life. (From Webster & Poulos, 1989)

As suggested earlier, the basic problem reported by the clients was self-defeating self-talk. Based on the sport psychology literature, I came to distinguish among 1) negative or **ineffective self-talk**, 2) positive or **more-effective self-talk**, and 3) **less-effective self-talk**. Table 1, taken from the

1   This manual can be ordered in an e-book format from the Institute for Stuttering Treatment and Research of the University Alberta. Information is available at https://marketplace.ualberta.ca/products/manual-facilitating-fluency

Webster and Poulos (1989) manual, summarizes the **characteristics** and **consequences** of the three types of self-talk.

Table 1: A Summary of Characteristics and Consequences of Self-Talk.
(From Webster & Poulos, 1989)

Self-Talk (ST) is about: Ourselves
Speech
Other people
Social and speaking situations

Ineffective S-T	Less-Effective S-T	More-Effective S-T
*Expresses hopelessness and helplessness	*Reminders of things not to do	*Reminders of skills over which we have control
*Intolerant of self and others	*Emphasis on how things could be better	*Action-oriented
*Self-critical	*Self-critical tone	*Focused and specific
*Negative	*Negative phrasing	*Positive
*Vague and general	*Unrealistic	*Realistic

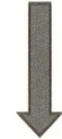 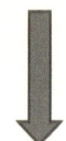 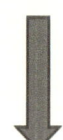

*Interferes with use of fluency skills	*Does not help or impede use of fluency skills	*Supports use of fluency skills
*Promotes apprehension		*Helps and supports communication activities
*Discourages communication activities		

Negative and ineffective self-talk actually interferes with entering social and speaking situations and interferes with even trying to use fluency skills. For example, if I were about to enter a social situation and find myself saying to myself that "My fluency skills have never worked in this situation. I'm just too tense," the prospects of using those skills and achieving success are remote. Just like with PFSP speech mechanics in which we want to replace movements that lead to stuttering with movements that lead to fluency, we want to replace ineffective self-talk with more-effective self-talk. In our example, that more-effective self-talk might be to say something specific, concrete, action-oriented, and positive like, "This is a great opportunity to practice my fluency skills, and I'm going to focus on using just full-breath to get started." This supports entering the situation; it supports being reminded of fluency skills; it guides what will be done; it provides a realistic sense of control.

There are things I could say that may not interfere with using fluency skills but which, because they are vague, do not facilitate use of fluency skills. For example, "This situation will be a test to see if my fluency skills really work." There are no reminders here about what one can control. We called this **less-effective self-talk**. When we recognize such self-talk being used, we need try to change it to **more-effective self-talk**.

More-effective self-talk is **not** saying general and positive self-affirmations to oneself like, "I can do it," or "I'm confident," or "I'll knock their socks off with this presentation," or "Saying this person's name will be easy," or "I am amazing." These are not substitutes for learning and using motoric fluency skills. **More-effective self-talk** is all about **reminding** ourselves of things over which we can have control and reminding ourselves why and how we should use fluency skills.

Table 2, which is at the end of the book in the Appendix Tables, provides examples of more-effective self-talk, less-effective self-talk, and ineffective self-talk in four different speaking contexts:
- Preparing for speaking situations that may evoke anxiety
- Coping when speech anxiety starts to build
- Coping when speech anxiety starts to overwhelm
- Coping when it's all over and the anxiety has passed

The examples in table 2 will be particularly relevant and meaningful to the reader who has experienced some stuttering treatment that has included acquiring fluency skills. This is simply because a lot of the emphasis in the examples is on reminders to use fluency skills over which we can have control and the use of which will facilitate fluent speech.

Typical situations which are difficult for people trying to use fluency skills consistently are ones involving time pressure, meeting family and friends with whom there may be a long history of speaking, and continuing to avoid words that are potentially problematic. Table 3, which also is at the end of the book in the Appendix Tables, includes a brief vignette around each kind of situation. Before you look at the self-talk or inappropriate thoughts associated with each vignette, imagine the ineffective self-talk or inappropriate thoughts the person described might have had that would lead to their reluctance to use fluency skills. Compare your answers to what is in the table. Stuttering treatment clients actually generated the statements in this table based on their experiences. Which self-talk statements in the table do you think would be particularly meaningful to you if you were in each situation? Can you think of other alternative statements? When doing this, just remember the characteristics of more-effective, less-effective, and ineffective self-talk.

A significant focus of the *Facilitating Fluency* manual deals with replacing ineffective with more-effective self-talk, but there are other sections dealing with managing tension (through techniques of progressive relaxation) in social and speaking situations, attacking avoidances (the why and how to avoid avoidances in speaking), and refining social skills (through learning and using social scripts). Other sections deal with managing daily practice of fluency skills, managing a structured diary, and managing the ups and downs of speech. These are all areas that would be covered in most stuttering treatment programs. I am delighted that this manual is still available these many years later.

* * * * * * * *

Throughout this time, the Ottawa Hospital Rehabilitation Centre supported an active alumni self-help group comprised largely of graduates of the program from over several years. Although the meetings were held at the Rehabilitation Centre and were overseen by a speech-language pathologist, they were truly "self-help." The group met on two or three weekends a year, and this provided opportunities for the graduates, recent and not-so-recent, to refresh with one another their use of fluency or stuttering modification skills (depending on what their therapy had been).

Among other things, the sessions also provided a safe venue to practice speaking with one another using fluency skills deliberately, to make brief speeches using their skills, to share experiences that they had either with their stuttering or with their use of fluency skills in their everyday life, and to provide friendship and support to one another. Some of the self-help group participants also participated in community-based programs like Toastmasters™ and occasional regional self-help meetings that gave them yet other opportunities to practice speaking in public.

I attended as many self-help weekends as I could, occasionally speaking at them, but far more often just listening and learning. Not every participant was a graduate of this program, and that was not a problem. Those non-graduate participants may have been to private practice therapists or to programs in other cities (including programs that had a different focus like "stuttering modification" or "easy stuttering"), and other participants had never had therapy and were there simply to learn from others about stuttering. So, not all participants shared the same approach to managing their speech. But what they (we) all had in common was that we were people who stuttered and who wanted to improve our speech, communication, and social skills, and that was empowering.

Participating in these groups, both the structured PFSP therapy groups and the self-help groups, very much benefitted my own speech. I found that over time I had picked up by osmosis and deliberate practice a version of the PFSP targets that I found helpful, especially the full breath and gentle onset targets. In retrospect, I'm sure the fluency skills I developed were not as ingrained or as well done as they would have been if I had gone through the program as a client and systematically worked through the exercises. However, I did try to incorporate what I had into my everyday speech, including my teaching at the university. That said, in retrospect I do regret about not having enrolled in the program as a client and done more structured "doing" rather than just "thinking and talking."

* * * * * * * *

In anticipation of Part III, which gets into strategies for managing speech, one further issue I need to raise is: **Is stuttering inevitable?** Over the years, I have met many individuals who stutter, all of whom are unique yet share many similarities in how their stuttering presents and how they elect to manage it. Despite these similarities, individuals often respond differently to scientific knowledge that demonstrates that stuttering has its origins in the brain. Some are pleased to learn that their stuttering is linked to biological/neurological origins, and is not attributable to something that they, their parents, or their teachers did or did not do. In contrast, others are distressed to learn that their stuttering has a biological/neurological origin that includes "areas of activation/deactivation" in the brain" during speaking or "anomalous wiring of the brain." Regardless of whether an individual is pleased or distressed to learn of the biological/neurological basis of stuttering, the fact remains that **biological does not mean inevitable** even if the brain is involved. Stuttering does not have to be an insurmountable life-long barrier; stuttering does not have to define a person; stuttering can be managed. **Managed does not mean cured**; it means there can be control over when disfluencies occur, how often or frequently they occur, and how impactful they are on communication and self-esteem. This is the theme of much of the rest of this book.

We are all familiar with the idea that the brain is the origin of behaviour, thought and emotions. What may not be so familiar with is the idea that behaviour, thought, and emotions can be the origin or guide of brain activity. If I ask you to imagine yourself sitting on a beach in the sunshine and you say you have conjured up that image, you have voluntarily changed your brain activity. The simple takeaway from this admittedly trivial example is that you and I have considerably greater control over our brains than we often credit ourselves with. I would suggest that, when we, as people who stutter, use cognitive strategies like self-talk, we can actually control left hemisphere activity, an idea introduced in chapter 6. Specifically, when we can voluntarily control our speech through monitoring, regulating speech rate, controlling beathing and voice onsets, **feeling** the movements associated with vocalizations, and being deliberate (and motorically organized) in our speech movements to maximize kinesthetic feedback (these are all components of most adult stuttering treatment programs), the act of doing these things will have the effect of altering left hemisphere SMA activity so it supports fluent speech.

I would similarly suggest that when we voluntarily control our fears and apprehensions about speaking by using techniques like progressive relaxation and more-effective self-talk, and when we systematically go into feared situations so we become less fearful, we are **doing** things that lower our right hemisphere activation. And when we control the right hemisphere activation, we minimize interference on the left hemisphere SMA, and we minimize stuttering.

This is all to say that when we use techniques and skills to control our speech and to control our thoughts and emotions, we are using techniques to control our brains in ways that can mitigate our inborn wiring anomalies to one degree or another. In fact, we may do more than that. The concept of **neuroplasticity**, the changeability of neuronal connections through experience, is well accepted today in the neurosciences. What it means is that, in principle and within limits, there is every reason to believe and expect that as people who stutter learn new fluency skills and apply them **consistently**, the wiring of the brain will modify and solidify so the new patterns of brain activity become more **embedded** and **automatic**. A hint of this possibility with stuttering was suggested in my earlier reference in chapter 5 to a 40-year-old electrophysiological study by Boberg et al. (1983) demonstrating a reduction in right hemisphere activation following stuttering treatment. What was not addressed in that study was whether the change was short- or long-term.

Although making a distinction between the "hardware" and "software" of the brain comes easily for those in the world of computers, that distinction does not work well when it comes to brain function. In 1949, the Canadian neuropsychologist, Dr. Donald Hebb, who was referenced earlier in various contexts, proposed a principle of how neural connections change and adapt with use, a principle that is still influential today in the neurosciences and in the development of artificial intelligence. The principle is,

> When an axon of cell A is near enough to excite cell B and repeatedly or persistently takes part in firing it, some growth process or metabolic change takes place in one or both cells such that A's efficiency, as one of the cells firing B, is increased. (Hebb, 1949, p. 62).

Using techniques and skills to control our thoughts and emotions not only allows us to control our immediate brain activity, as suggested above, but it also allows us to change on-going and longer-term neuronal patterns of activity in our brains (i.e., learning). Hebb's principle implies that this change involves neither hardware alone nor software alone, but probabilistic "brainware."

PART III

Putting it All Together: Strategies for Managing Speech

CHAPTER 8

From University Neuroscientist to University Administrator

I n 1991, my career as an academic changed directions from having had a focus on teaching and research to having a primary focus on university leadership and administration. That new focus required my speaking frequently in many new and varied contexts, something I both welcomed (in principle) and feared (in practice). This provided opportunities to put into practice what I had been learning through my research, reading, and my frequent interactions with people who stutter. The purpose of this chapter is **not** to describe what I did or accomplished **professionally** in each new leadership role. Instead, it is about what I learned and accomplished **personally** in dealing with my speech and its management in these roles.

The trajectory for this leadership role began some years earlier with my appointment as department chair at Carleton University, as I introduced in chapter 4. Early on, I quickly came to realize several things about speaking and stuttering that I needed to work on if I were to become a credible department chair.

First, social scripts. Perhaps because I had avoided or just stood back from social interaction over the years, or because I had focused so much on **not stuttering** when in social and professional situations, my knowledge and understanding of the usual social scripts that we all follow in our everyday lives was weak. There were many situations in which I did not have a clear idea of **what** I should be saying, **when**, and **to whom** I should say it, or what I should be **doing**. For example, I had to learn how to introduce myself and others in different social and professional contexts; how and when to shake hands; the importance of maintaining eye contact when speaking; how to graciously thank a colleague for doing something for me; how to lead and actively participate in a small meeting of two or three people in my office; how to end a meeting with a summary of understandings; how to make the many different kinds of phone calls that arise in a week; how to move through a reception; and the list goes on. I certainly had some idea of how to do these things, but I wasn't comfortable, I wasn't practiced, and the scripts did not come automatically. I felt self-conscious. So, I started doing a lot of observing of others who I thought would be good role models, followed by notetaking of things that were said and done. I found it helpful to occasionally review those notes and deliberately find opportunities to practice particular social scripts. The more I engaged in these kinds of activities, the more comfortable, skilled, and confident I felt doing them, and the less inclined I was to avoid or withdraw from them (remember what the motivation to withdraw does to right hemisphere activation). But there are some social scripts with which I never got particularly comfortable.

The social script issue was particularly acute for me with respect to answering and speaking on the phone. As you, the reader, may have gathered from earlier chapters, I had always avoided using the phone. Now I found that when the phone rang on my desk, the sense of impending loss of control would instantly flood my mind and interfere with my remembering what I would want to say when I pick up the receiver. I needed a script, and that could be just a small note I placed in front of the phone with the words to say. Then I could focus quickly on my breathing and using a gentle voice onset. Equally as difficult was making a phone call because, after putting off making the call for as long as possible (and becoming increasingly anxious the whole time), I had three things to remember to say: to whom I wanted to speak, my name, and why I was calling. Word substitution was not an option.

Second, I had been too preoccupied my whole life with **how** I was saying things rather than on the what and **why** of speaking, and that was where careful preparation on content became helpful. But preparation was time consuming. Also, I dreaded meetings that started with round-table introductions. By the end of the introductions, I never remembered anyone's name because I was so focused on how I was going to say my own name when my turn came. To deal with that, I would often offer to start the round of introductions. That way, I would get my own name out before the anxiety started to build, and I could then focus on attending to the names of others at the table. By taking the lead, I found myself feeling more in control of everything, including my speech.

Similarly, when I was in committee meetings, I often found that being preoccupied with my speech or with that pervasive sense of impending loss of control, could distract me from keeping track of where the meeting was going, what I wanted to say on certain agenda items, and the order in which I wanted to make points. Having an annotated agenda prepared before the meeting with a list of key points associated with each agenda item helped me to keep my thoughts organized when it was time to speak. As a result, speech stayed more under control. I also found that offering to take the minutes of the meeting helped me with attending to what others were saying and remembering details that I thought were important. It was a matter of focussing on others, not on myself.

Third, I quickly began to realize as I started my department chair role that it is not shameful to stutter nor to openly disclose that I stutter. Open disclosure would ensure that stuttering did not become the "elephant in the room." A matter-of-fact disclosure could be made easily in a one-on-one conversation with someone who didn't know I stutter, with a small group, or indeed with a large audience. Doing so meant that when a hesitation or block might occur, no "secret" was being disclosed. Being open also presented an occasional opportunity for education of others about the nature of stuttering. Our non-stuttering friends and colleagues are interested in stuttering, and there is no shortage of good questions out there just waiting to be asked by them and answered by us. A little encouragement to ask is appreciated by the curious.

Becoming the department chair provided a tremendous learning and maturing experience for me, and it started me down a university leadership path. As I discuss later in this chapter, that path led ultimately to deanships at two universities, and I became director of a speech and hearing university program. These roles pushed me, as I had been pushed in earlier days by teachers and my mother, into speaking situations that I would have previously avoided at almost all costs. However, I came to realize in this role that there was no inevitable contradiction between being a person who stutters and being an **effective leader**.

The good news for the person who stutters, like me, is that effective leadership is more about a lot of **good listening** than about a lot of talking. A speech-language pathologist friend of mine, Ms. Jill Harrison, once commented that "people who stutter are often too preoccupied to listen or listen well." And a good listener does not just sit quietly, daydream, or drift off when others are talking; a good listener is mentally engaged in listening; asking questions internally if not externally; making eye contact with the speaker; responding with occasional nonverbal gestures that convey understanding and interest; and occasionally offering an opinion or comment. It took a while for me to learn that as a department chair. Although a person who stutters may or may not be an introvert, perhaps the value of good listening to leadership is one reason that Susan Cain, author of *Quiet: The Power of Introverts in a World that Can't Stop Talking*, cited research that indicates that the vast majority of CEOs of major corporations are introverts. They listen.

Being **well-prepared** for meetings and social interactions helped me listen. I did not have to constantly focus on what I might say and how I would say it; I could be a far more active and engaged listener which in turn facilitated fluent speech. Being prepared for interaction seemed to keep the conversation slower, unrushed, and "non-competitive." If being prepared meant I wasn't preoccupied, not only could I listen better but also I could be more measured in my responses and comments. In fact, I began to learn as a department chair that good active listening is the key to working successfully with faculty members, regardless of whether or not one is a person who stutters. As will be clear later, I still had a lot to learn about that active-listening concept when I arrived at Brock University some years later.

Another piece of good news for the person who stutters, especially who has received therapy in a program that focusses on controlled speech motor movements, is that persuasive speaking is not about a lot of **fast** talking. My observation has been that regardless of whether or not they are persons who stutter, the best speakers who are interesting and influential in what they say generally speak slowly and deliberately, with pauses as appropriate, so their listeners can absorb what is being said. As I have raised earlier, **slow and deliberate articulation** can also facilitate fluency in people who stutter because it can enhance kinesthetic information to the brain which is important for guiding oral muscle movements. Slower speaking can also provide a little more time to organize thoughts and fluency skills (both motoric and emotional). That said, I know that some therapy graduates still feel that their speech sounds unnaturally slow when they are using fluency skills. I've always been impressed at what a good friend an audio recorder can be to remind one that the new slower and deliberate speech is not slower than the **old speech** filled with hesitations, repetitions, and blockages. It is also not much slower than that of many effective speakers who do not stutter.

The most difficult speaking situation I encountered while department chair at Carleton occurred when I was required to lead a memorial service for a well-respected colleague in the department who had taken his own life under tragic circumstances. This was an emotionally charged situation for everyone, and the service attracted many colleagues from across the campus. Obviously, I was anxious that the event and my speaking role in it would go well. Some months earlier, by happy coincidence, I had decided to learn about progressive relaxation as a means of releasing muscle tension and feelings of stress. Sitting to the side of the room before the proceedings got underway afforded me an opportunity to practice the simple exercises quietly. It made a difference. Going through the steps of voluntarily tensing and relaxing different muscle groups and then just feeling the relaxation also served as a most effective distraction from that otherwise pervasive sense of impending loss of control. These exercises blocked ineffective self-talk like, "my speech is going to be terrible because I am so tense." And it wasn't. The speech I gave was difficult, but I was more in control than usual. As I looked back on the time, I think that experiencing that voluntary control over my body tension helped me to exert voluntary control over my use of fluency skills (related to breathing, slower speech, stretched sounds, smooth onset of sounds, etc.) and of more-effective self-talk. And of course, all was well prepared in advance with no words left to chance. I simply had to focus on slow and deliberate reading and saying what was on the page in front of me, thinking of the content mainly to influence where I put pauses and emphasis, and glancing occasionally at the audience. No one expected me to speak extemporaneously, and none of the other speakers that day spoke without reading notes. I became a convert to the power of progressive relaxation and the use of more-effective self-talk in difficult speaking situations.

Many of the substantive issues I faced as a new department chair were ones that I thought could be mitigated through the development of department approved policies and procedures and implemented by me with collaboration, fairness, and transparency. I felt I could provide the required leadership. The bullying issues that were part of the department's disfunction at the time were potentially more difficult.

My approach to the development of department policies and procedures fit well with being someone who stutters. I relied on **writing** (was avoidance continuing to thrive?). I was aware of the different perspectives on issues in the department, augmented of course by conversations with colleagues. My approach was to draft a position paper that acknowledged the different perspectives on the issue or problem that the policy was intended to address, gave some history, and proposed a reasonable policy and set of procedures based on articulated and explicit principles. I then brought that to a department meeting for consideration, revision, and approval. Because my position on the issue was generally clear in what I had written, I did not have to speak much to advance that position; other colleagues would speak for me if necessary. And because the entirety of my position was out there, I didn't feel I needed to rush in making some particular point out of fear I would forget the next point or because I felt I needed to put my particular point into a broader context. Occasionally, if

I had not succeeded in capturing the prevailing sentiment in the department or there were new ideas that emerged from the discussions, I would repeat the process and prepare a fresh position paper for consideration. Over time, the culture of the department did change, and we experienced greatly improved civility, cooperation, and just plain fun. What I learned was people generally like to have background and forewarning about what they are going to be asked to discuss. They also need opportunities to be heard respectfully. When these are provided, particularly those related to respect, people can usually accept openly reached decisions with which they may disagree. More germane to the present discussion, I also learned that **clear and succinct writing** is an effective leadership tool for anyone, but particularly for someone who stutters. It doesn't replace speech but reduces complete reliance on speech and it can level the communication playing field in some circumstances.

I saw one of my important roles as an academic leader to be to promote and support and advocate for the scholarly activities and recognition of my colleagues, and I took a lot of satisfaction in that role. My colleagues' successes in the classroom and the research lab were substantial, and I was frankly proud to be the chair of such a department. Providing that support required presentations by me in committee meetings at the Faculty and occasionally the university level, and in one-on-one discussions with the dean and other department chairs. I relied heavily on being well-prepared when I had to speak, and as I have indicated earlier, if I was prepared, I found I could be reasonably fluent. But preparation was key because I could not think well on my feet while struggling with what I wanted to say, with the order in which I wanted to say things, and with how I was going to say them. And as I have described elsewhere, preparation often required writing myself notes, which could range from a few jot notes on a file card to what amounted essentially to a script, to which I could refer if necessary. Depending on the context, I might even mark the script with where I should insert pauses or word emphasis. And, of course, I included my usual reminder at the top of the notes about breathing and stretching sounds and talking deliberately. Interestingly, I did not attract attention (at least that I was aware of) by having these notes, particularly in more formal meetings where others would have papers on the table and often consult them. I was not alone in being prepared.

Although speaking at large Faculty or university committee meetings presented its challenges, often one-on-one meetings would present their own unique challenges. I have long had the impression that in this more intimate and familiar context, the person with whom I would be talking would often start speaking far faster than they would have in a large or even small group setting. The challenge for me was that I found myself increasingly getting drawn into either speaking faster or feeling I should be speaking faster. That would heighten that sense of impending loss of control and generate anxiety (and probably increased right hemisphere activity). All I could do in that situation was to very deliberately slow down my own rate of speech which often in turn seemed to slow down (temporarily at least) the rate of speech of the other person. Doing this, and continuing to do this as needed, was harder than it might seem. I do find these interaction dynamics quite fascinating.

As my research and my involvement with the stuttering groups at the Rehabilitation Centre progressed, I developed new approaches to managing my speech, approaches I have alluded to earlier. Some involved **imagining** what was going on in my brain when I stuttered and what I could do to alter the balance of activity between the cerebral hemispheres. By the time my term as chair ended, my social skills were much stronger, and I was getting better at making introductions and unplanned off-the-cuff comments. I was also relying less on detailed notes and more on short and simple notes on a single file card which could remind me of the points I wanted to make and the order in which I might want to make them. The cards usually also contained just a word or two reminder of more-effective self-talk and of one or two fluency skills (like "stretch sounds," "exaggerate movements," etc.). To the extent it is feasible (and often it's not), I still rely on notes of what I want to say and the order in which I want to say it, especially when I am using the phone.

Another duty I took on as the department chair was to chair most of the graduate oral examinations in the department. Although time-consuming, there were a number of reasons for taking this on. First, it was a simple way for me to keep up with the details of the research programs of the faculty supervising graduate students and this helped me to be able to represent those programs in various venues. Second, it was a way for me to get to know the graduate students in the different research areas of the department. Third, it provided me with opportunities to speak in a controlled environment which involved a similar script for most examinations. As I have noted earlier, speech fluency improves with **repetition of a word or phrase**; it also improves with practiced social scripts. After repetition of the basic script in several exams, speech increasingly flowed easily from the tongue, usually relatively stutter-free. The fourth reason I chaired the exams was frankly negative. Concerns had been expressed to me about how some graduate students had been treated poorly in oral exams by some faculty members: favouritism, conflicts of interest, disrespect, and even occasional bullying. So, I decided to chair most exams, lay out in written form the ground-rules for the procedures, and write the decisions and recommendations myself. It was my expectation that my presence and involvement as department chair would cut off inappropriate behaviour. It did. And I got to know the students and the faculty better, and I gained a lot of speaking experience in chairing those examination committee meetings and mediating differences of opinion on thesis modifications to be required.

Despite the rewards and satisfactions, I found that two terms in an administrative and leadership role that involved so much speaking and chairing meetings was wearing. At the end of the second term, I felt ready to return to being a regular faculty member. I believe that when I stepped down from the chair position, I left the department in better shape than when I had started, and I left it well-positioned for the future. I also believe most of my colleagues would have agreed. Although I had some conflicts with a few faculty members who wanted to act like free agents rather than as university colleagues, over time most of them did come around. At the end of my term, the informal leader of that group conceded that I had done a good job, almost as good as he would have done himself. Interestingly, I never encountered any overt negative comments about my speech from any of that small group. They were decent people, but they were also very wise.

I was satisfied with what I had done as chair, particularly as a person who stutters. I also felt that because of that role, my speech, my skills, and my confidence in speaking were far better than they had been previously. The position pushed me to speak in so many contexts and to figure out how to speak better and how not to avoid speaking. And then, as ironic as this may be, at the end of my seven years as chair, I found that my appetite had been whetted, at least in principle, to think occasionally about pursuing a decanal or provost role. Being in the centre of things was energizing, and I continued to be interested in how an academic administrator and leader can, in the context of faculty academic freedom and budgetary limitations, facilitate the enhancement of the learning experience of undergraduate students. But for the time being, my return to more classroom teaching and my evolving research studies and group work with stuttering clients at the Rehabilitation Centre were sufficiently satisfying to keep me well occupied and focused. I had no interest in actually moving on at the time.

At the end of my term as department chair, I was pleased to start a much-needed six-month sabbatical leave and I decided to include in my leave activities a non-credit course in oral French offered through the school board. My stuttering was not kind to me in that course. Although I had always been able to read and write French reasonably well from my high school days in Montreal, I simply could not seem to process the sounds of spoken foreign languages nor produce the sounds in French except for occasional short well-practiced phrases. The phrase that for some bizarre reason still sticks in my mind and that would roll easily off the tongue was, "Mais, oui, je parle français très couramment," meaning, "yes, I speak French very fluently." That was my only phrase and so it didn't lead anywhere except awkward silence. I refrained from using it much. In my French class I tried, I really did try, but my stuttering was terrible despite all the relaxation and self-talk adjustments and brain imaging I could muster. For the speech assignments, I had to write them fully and then read them, just as I had done in English for some committee meetings at Carleton. That's not what oral French is supposed to be. I have now reluctantly accepted with some personal dissatisfaction that I am not and will never be a bilingual Canadian.

* * * * * * * *

While on my sabbatical leave, I also broadened my speaking experiences outside the university by volunteering to serve on the Ottawa-Carleton Regional District Health Council. The role of council which reported to the provincial government, was to identify health priorities for the region. Probably influenced by my background in psychology, I was asked to chair the Mental Health Committee of the council, and it was an interesting time to do so because of the growing emphasis on moving the care and treatment of people with mental illness from hospitals to the community. I had not understood that the council expected that the key activity of my committee for the coming year was to lead a broad community consultation on the needs of people with mental illness in the community. That might involve considerable public speaking. My immediate inclination, of course, was to avoid situations like this, but as was invariably the case in the past, being pushed into the situation and accepting it had a positive and empowering outcome. Fortunately for me, much of the required speaking at the public community consultations was done by staff and paid facilitators who led the sessions. But I did find that the more I contributed to these sessions and the more I applied what I had been learning about reducing interference and facilitating fluency, the easier public speaking became. It could even be fun!

For the next few years as a regular faculty member, I also took on more university-based responsibilities that required speaking and mediating in a variety of conflict contexts. For example, the vice-president and provost asked me to chair a review committee concerned with the School of Architecture and, specifically, with aspects of its culture that were problematic with respect to the evaluation of student projects. I agreed to do so. Committee meetings, interviews with students and faculty, and public presentations all kept my fluency skills honed. I was also asked to chair the search committee for a new Director of the School of Social Work at a time when the school was facing major divisions within it. These divisions were largely ideologically based and not dissimilar to those found at the time at other schools of social work across Canada. Of course, what brought the school factions together, at least temporarily, was unhappiness that an "outsider" would be chairing the search for their new director. Again, this provided lots of opportunities to practice controlled speaking and more-effective self-talk. I enjoyed these assignments because they greatly broadened my view of the university and contributed to my record of experiences that later made me an attractive candidate for leadership positions elsewhere. They are further examples of how I benefitted once again by being encouraged into new roles that required speaking.

In early 1991, I received an e-mail from an old friend from McGill days whom I had not seen for twenty-five years. I was aware that she had completed her PhD and had established a strong reputation for herself in her field. She said she had recently been elected president of a national organization and was going to be in Ottawa for meetings the following week. She wondered if we might have dinner one night when she would be in town. It was one of those unpredicted and pivotal events that would change the direction of my life.

I accepted the invitation. When we met, we talked in broad strokes about our careers and in particular about the joys and challenges of university administration. She shared with me that she had recently been offered the position of Dean of the Faculty of Social Sciences at Brock University in St. Catharines, Ontario. Although she thought the position was interesting and she was well received in her interview, she had just decided to decline the offer for various personal reasons. She went on to say that if I was looking for a change and if this was the kind of position in which I might be interested, she would pass my name on to the search consultant.

As I thought about the position during and after that dinner, I realized that I was ready for change. Twenty-plus years can be a long time in one workplace: basically, the same people, same issues, same environment, similar teaching, similar research grants, same conflicts. While I came to see that I was ready for change, I had not realized that until then; and of course I had done nothing to even explore a possible change. Two or three years earlier, I had applied for the position of Dean of the Faculty of Social Sciences at Carleton, but another candidate was appointed. She was a good choice. In retrospect, I realize now that I needed more change than would have been provided with a new position and title at Carleton. It did not take much thought for me to realize that the readiness was there, and I didn't need arm-twisting or convincing to at least explore what a change would involve. I heard from the search consultant a few days later.

Interestingly, despite the speaking challenges I had as a department chair, I had no hesitation I can remember about whether I could deal with the greater speaking commitments that I knew would go along with being a dean. I must have just assumed I could do it, as I had dealt with these types of commitments as a department chair. I realized that Brock University could not have been a better fit. It was a university similar to Carleton but newer and smaller, and aspiring to become a comprehensive university. Its psychology department, part of the Faculty of Social Sciences, had a good number of excellent faculty members with an applied focus, which I found attractive and which I think attracted the Brock faculty to me. I also expected, somewhat naïvely it turned out, that I would continue my research program at Brock if I were to move there. I accepted the offer to be dean, effective July 1, 1991.

Brock University

At the time, Brock University was a comparatively small liberal arts and science university which prided itself on quality undergraduate teaching achieved through small classes and a tutorial system. I quickly realized there were the beginnings of an intergenerational conflict whereby the roles of teaching and research in the academy were under scrutiny. As was the case at Carleton, many of the older faculty members had come to Brock to establish the university through undergraduate teaching; and many of the more recently appointed faculty were committed to their personal research aspirations. Like at Carleton, this was fuel for simmering conflict that occasionally overflowed into other issues.

I took my research equipment with me to Brock intending to continue my research. I was planning to focus on kinesthetic guidance of movement by people who stutter. I had not fully appreciated the implications of no longer having Joanne Hakkaku as my research assistant, and not having the Ottawa Hospital Rehabilitation Centre close by as a magnet for people who stutter. Unfortunately, in the fall of 1991, Marie Poulos was killed in a car accident just south of Ottawa. Her death was a huge loss to the fluency community and impacted my research momentum. However, my inability to continue my research program mainly reflected the fact that being a dean of a large Faculty with a dozen departments and programs was all-consuming. I was able to keep up with reading the research literature in the area, and I was able to continue to attend some conferences, but new experiments were off the table.

From the start, I found I had more frequent public presentations than I had had at Carleton, and I continued my long-standing practice of including two speech strategies into those presentations. First, I continued to write down at the top of my notes a brief reminder to take a controlled breath, stretch my sounds, speak slowly, exaggerate oral movements, and start sounds gently. I usually didn't have to refer to the notes, but this reminder in front of me was always there if I needed help to start the presentation with control, regardless of what distractions there may have been in the room at the moment. I always found that starting slowly and deliberately put my left hemisphere into gear, so to speak, after which I did not have to consciously focus as much on the self-talk controls, but they were still there written at the top of a page if I needed them.

I should add that there have been times when the approach I just described did not work well, and almost always those occasions were ones when I was coming down with a head-cold and not feeling well. Despite my trying to focus and to exaggerate oral movements, the movements and breathing just wouldn't come together in a coordinated manner. Even just trying to formulate what I might want to say was particularly difficult. So, all I could do was accept the situation, minimize speaking, and, if appropriate, comment about the situation in a low-key manner. And get some extra sleep. Others seemed to understand. Managing speech doesn't mean eliminating stuttering in all circumstances; managing simply means using the skills and inner resources at hand and not feeling badly at the end.

My second practice, which I have alluded to earlier, relates to being open about stuttering. I came to start many public presentations (although not the ceremonial ones involving my reading of the names of graduates at convocation, as I will discuss later) by saying something like,

> I'm delighted to be here today. Thank you for inviting me. Before I get started, I thought I would share with you that I am a person who stutters, and you may see some good demonstrations of stuttering this morning. But maybe you won't. I have stuttered all my life. Usually my speech

is pretty good, and I expect that today will be one of those days, but sometimes I can get hung up on a word or a phrase. If that happens, please bear with me. It's nothing to be concerned about. Just so you know.

If my presentation was to be about stuttering research or treatment, this kind of disclosure served as a good segue into the content. For me, the value of disclosure is that it reduces anxiety about stuttering in front of a group, and according to the Two-Factor Interference Model, it does that by reducing right hemisphere activation as a source of interference with my speech. The audience knows I stutter, and they may get a first-hand experience of my stuttering. So, I thought, if I have a block or repetitions, it's no big deal, I don't feel vulnerable because I have already disclosed, and my right hemisphere stays calm. If that hemisphere remains calm, I would tell myself, it doesn't interfere with my left SMA, and that in turn helps me organize the motor movements and fully use the kinesthetic cues I need for fluent speech. At least that is how I would see it.

I had done very much the same thing in the initial meeting of my classes each term when I was actively teaching at Carleton. I felt it served to clear the air and removed questions. Interestingly, I would often have one or two students come up to me after that class or sometimes after a later class, just to tell me they or friends or family members stutter and appreciated that I had disclosed that I stutter. Of course, even if I hadn't disclosed my stuttering, students would have become aware of it within the first five minutes of class. However, I suspect that without my disclosure I would not have heard from the students about their experiences. Being open gave permission to others to be open. I thought it better just to get the stuttering out there so there would be no surprise or speculation.

I used these strategies when heading off to Nijmegen in the Netherlands for a conference on stuttering and speech motor control at which I had been invited to make a presentation on my research. What complicated things was that, in a brief moment of mutual insanity, my now-spouse, Anne Godden-Webster, and I decided that she should accompany me to the conference with our two young children in tow (one was not quite three years old, and the other was just over one year). Baby formula having leaked onto my presentation slides, a fussy child, limited sleep at night, a badly crushed tie, and a lost doll at the hotel did not facilitate fluent speech for my presentation. I was pleased the proceedings were published afterwards (Webster, 1997), because I remember nothing of my presentation or the presentations of others. This was one of the experiences that led me to realize that, with a young family, my days of conducting new research studies and contributing papers to conferences were numbered, at least for the time being.

In the following year, however, I did accept two back-to-back invitations to speak in the UK and again in Europe. Anne and the children did not travel with me. The first, a three-day workshop in Aahlborg, Denmark, started on the morning that Princess Diana was killed in a car accident in Paris. Her tragic death was so sudden and shocking, we all had trouble focusing on the workshop. Needless to say, issues of fluency and brain function were not at the forefront of mind for most of the participants. The second invitation was for an address at the annual meeting of the British Stammering Association. My session was scheduled to be at the same time as Princess Diana's funeral. I was re-scheduled for later that day but for only half the original allocated time. After some scrambling to re-organize the talk, rewrite and expand my self-talk notes, and refresh my progressive relaxation exercises, I gave what I believe was a credible presentation. Needless to say, there was limited attention focused on what I might have had to say. So much for my international jet-setting presentations while at Brock.

In thinking about my stuttering experiences at Brock University, I wanted to start with the most challenging duty required of me as a dean who stutters: reading the names of the graduates in my Faculty at convocation. For readers who may not have been at a university, graduands (a graduand is the student who is about to become a graduate) receive their diplomas in a formal ceremony called convocation. The faculty and senior administrators don colourful gowns, hoods, and often hats of various shapes and sizes (some liken it all to emulating peacocks) and the graduands, wearing gowns, hoods, and mortar board hats, are called individually to the stage to have their degree conferred by the chancellor. It really is a grand and very happy occasion. Except for a dean who stutters.

The job of the dean was to present each graduand by name to the chancellor and the audience. At Brock, students came to the stage in pairs, and each student would give the dean a card on which their name was printed, along with the names of any special awards they were receiving. The dean's job was simply to read the names and awards, and the students would then progress across the stage to the chancellor. There was no avoiding this duty. There was also no avoiding the script for the dean to read which started with, "Mr. Chancellor, I have the honour to present…" even if the dean has difficulties getting m-words started, as I do. Also, there is no substituting an "easier-to-say name" for a "more-difficult-to-say" name. The student, Megan, is "Megan," and saying "Samantha" because s-sounds are easier for me than m-sounds just doesn't cut it for the graduate whose name is Megan. One can practice the names ahead of time using the program, but because not all students whose names are on the program actually show up, and because some students get themselves out of alphabetical order, the program is of limited help for the actual occasion. The dean has to rely on the cards carried by the graduands.

During my years at Brock, the university was becoming increasingly multicultural with students from all around the world, and the deans' challenge, which all the deans took seriously, was to use the correct pronunciation of the names. My approach was typical. If in doubt about the pronunciation of an unfamiliar name on the graduand list, I could usually find someone in the university with experience in the language who could help ahead of time. Then, at convocation, when the students approached my podium with their cards, I could usually figure out the probable origin of the name, quickly use a pencil to break the name into syllables, mark on the card which syllable(s) probably should have emphasis, and note in some way the probable pronunciation of the different letter combinations in one or more syllables. After that, I would just say into the microphone each of the two graduand names (and any awards), using the appropriate syllabic pronunciation and emphasis, while remembering to speak slowly and deliberately, starting with a controlled breath and voice onset, and adding a bit of prosodic emphasis on the last syllable to convey some excitement about the achievement. After the first six or eight pairs of names, a rhythm would set in, and everything would flow more easily and smoothly.

Although reading the names at convocation presented challenges to me as a person who stutters, I always got through it without catastrophe, and I always felt wonderful to be part of such an important day in the lives our students. Convocation truly is the highlight in the university year. That said, I was always so glad to see the end of the line of graduands!

There are dangers with the kind of analysis I have just described. The experience that I remember most vividly is of a graduand who had a seemingly simple first name. I remember my analysis went roughly as follows:

> Eastern European in origin. First syllable was **Ja** having a **Ya** sound. Second syllable was a **nay** sound. Emphasis probably on the first syllable. First name is pronounced, **Ya-Nay**, add the last name, and say the whole name into the microphone.

As I read her name and she walked by my podium, she muttered, "I've never been called *that* before." It was only later, after I sat down, that I realized to my horror that I had indeed mispronounced her first name. If you think of this name as in fact having just a single syllable, J-a-n-e, you will understand that somewhere in Canada there is a Brock graduate whose name was butchered by her dean.

In chapter 2, I commented very briefly on using writing to avoid speaking and that this avoidance method got me into difficulty at various points in my administrative history. Early in my years as a dean, I learned that writing and speaking are not the same, and there are many situations in which the written word serves to complicate and escalate rather than simplify and resolve issues.

Part way through my term as dean at Brock, I was faced with a situation in which I realized there were marked inequities among the faculty members with respect to their teaching workloads. I wanted to address this by asking faculty who were not engaged in significant research activities to take on more undergraduate teaching duties than faculty members who had research programs supported by grants, were publishing that research, and were supervising graduate students. I made the mistake of relying on the written word rather than the spoken word in the initial communication with the few affected faculty. In retrospect, I am sure some avoidance of speaking was involved in my decision to write, but in fairness to myself, I thought at the time that some formality was required. I learned that, at least in the first instance, nothing beats the personal connection formed by the spoken word. I think now that, had I spoken individually with affected faculty members instead of writing to them, and had I used the good active listening skills I had tried to hone at Carleton, I could have negotiated reasonably amicably an understanding on their workload. Instead, writing escalated the situation in that it was perceived as threatening, and it allowed supporters of faculty unionization to seize on this as an example of what they might call the "uncaring and arbitrary actions of management that could only be resolved through a faculty union." One can debate whether unionization was ultimately good or bad for the university and the faculty, but my avoidance of speaking and relying on writing undoubtedly tipped the finely balanced scales at the time to unionization. I share this account as a caution to people who stutter that choosing to write instead of to speak, particularly in this day of texting and e-mails, may be a satisfying short term avoidance technique, but it can have longer term downsides one may regret. It's not just the ideas and words that matter; how they are communicated can make all the difference.

I was at Brock as a dean for two five-year terms. In my eleventh year at Brock, after my decanal contract had ended, I started a year of administrative leave. This type of leave, not unusual at Canadian universities, is offered to members of the senior administration who are ending their terms. It is similar to, but technically different from, a sabbatical leave. Its purpose could include giving the individual an opportunity to get their research or teaching work up to speed again before rejoining the faculty, or even to look for a new position at another university. My family and I thought it would be an interesting experience to visit for five months a university in New Zealand with the goal of reactivating my research program to prepare for my return. By September, planning for the visit was well advanced. However, the year was 2001, and in September the world experienced 9-11, which impacted everyone including former deans on administrative leave. Travel would have to wait until the world settled down.

A few weeks after 9-11, I was approached out of the blue by an audiologist friend at the School of Communication Sciences and Disorders of the

University of Western Ontario in London, Ontario, asking me, on behalf of some of his colleagues, to consider applying for the position of school director. The school had two major professional and research programs, one in speech-language pathology and the other in audiology. The school was academically strong, and the research of some of the faculty at the time was well-known nationally and internationally. Adding to the school's lustre, it was home to the newly established National Center for Audiology.

However, the school was feeling the strain of internal relationship challenges and conflicts both between faculty members in the two programs and within the speech-language pathology program itself. It seems that one reason for the audiologists' interest in me as a potential director was that I was not part of either of the two professions, but still had a good understanding of each of their respective underlying disciplinary bases. I also was known to have had some success at Carleton and Brock (despite the unionization snafu) with being a mediator of internal conflicts, a promoter of civility, an advocate for students, and a facilitator for faculty to get on with their work. After some consideration, I recognized that it would probably be easier for me to reinstate and continue my research program on stuttering at Western than at Brock because of Western's professional school with a clinic and its stronger research ethos. Also, I was aware of the difficulties former deans often experience in returning to their home department as regular faculty members. This was especially so when the former dean had not previously been part of that department; that was my situation. So, I decided to go through the formal search process at Western, met with the faculty and the dean, and was offered the position of school director. Based on assurances about the resources I could expect for implementing a plan for dealing with the relationship issues facing the school, I accepted the offer effective July 1, 2002.

University of Western Ontario (now Western University)

Upon my arrival at Western, I was pleased to be encouraged by the dean and my new colleagues to reactivate my research on stuttering. I was provided with space and funds to purchase some updated equipment. The position was particularly helpful in getting me plugged into the speech-language pathology community, both in Ontario and nationally. As school director,

I served on a provincial committee of directors of schools of rehabilitation sciences, and on a national committee of directors of Canadian schools of speech-language pathology and audiology. Through this latter committee, I met Dr. Joy Armson, the director of the Dalhousie school. In the fall of 2003, Joy asked me to consider being a member of a panel being organized by her dean to review her school's programs and organization. I agreed to do this, never suspecting it would have pivotal future consequences that I will describe shortly.

By the end of my first year at Western, my lab was set up again and I had started to establish the networking connections that would be helpful in finding research participants. Based on the research I had done at Carleton with the initiation of finger movements, I started a study involving the initiation of complex oral movements (swallowing) in people who stutter in response to internal versus external response directions. I had a wonderful new research assistant, Bea Goffin and, as expected, it was somewhat easier to find research participants at Western than it had been at Brock. So, things started to move along well. Unfortunately, when we were almost finished testing participants in that first study and were starting to analyze the data, I realized to my horror that the logic of the experimental design was flawed and that I would not be able to draw any meaningful conclusions about oral response initiation in stutterers versus non-stutterers as I had planned. Normally I would have chalked this all up to experience, adjusted the procedures, found new participants, and started over again. However, my work environment was about to change.

By this time, I was becoming disenchanted with Western because the resources for the school that I had been promised were not forthcoming. Without those resources, the plan I had developed at the time of my appointment to deal with the internal conflicts in the school would not be feasible, and I saw little prospect for dealing with the issues effectively without those additional resources. And the personal and professional conflicts among the faculty, while under control, still made life in the school, for some, like walking on eggshells. I was 60 years of age and, in light of the circumstances, was no longer certain that I wanted to remain at Western until retirement.

It was at this point, a few months after I had participated on the program review panel at Dalhousie, I was contacted again by Dr. Joy Armson, the director of that school, this time to ask if I would be interested in putting my name forward for the position of Dean of the Dalhousie University Faculty of Health Professions. The dean had just announced her resignation, and a search had started for a replacement.

On the one hand, I was delighted to be asked. From my review of the Dalhousie school, I already knew a fair amount about it and the Faculty of Health Professions, and my impressions were highly positive. Given the size and complexity of that Faculty with its multitude and variety of health profession programs, I felt I was being presented with a wonderful opportunity to learn so much more than I knew about the health professions and health care, and potentially to have a meaningful impact in Nova Scotia through supporting health research and the preparation of future healthcare professionals.

On the other hand, I recognized that if I were to accept the position at Dalhousie, the move would probably mean the end of my active involvement in further research studies on stuttering. My duties as a dean at Dalhousie would be at least as all-consuming as they had been at Brock. As I thought about what research projects I would be foregoing, I realized that by this point I had already answered, at least as a first approximation, the two basic questions I had started with: What is different about the brains of people who stutter? And what underlies variability in stuttering severity in people who stutter?

After some struggle, I asked Joy to forward my name to her search committee and the search consultant. I was interviewed and when offered the position of dean, started negotiating my departure from Western. I must say that the administrators at Western were gracious and helpful in facilitating the transition after just three years. I started at Dalhousie in July, 2005.

Dalhousie University

Dalhousie University, in Halifax, Nova Scotia, is a mid-sized university in terms of student numbers but a large-sized university in terms of the range of programs it offers. The Faculty of Health Professions (now called the Faculty of Health) is one the three health-related faculties, the other two being medicine and dentistry. The Faculty of Health Professions is home for a wide range of professional programs including nursing, phys-iotherapy, occupational therapy, social work, speech-language pathology, audiology, kinesiology, pharmacy, health administration, health promo-tion, to name most. Although my administrative appointment was Dean of the Faculty of Health Professions, my academic appointment was in the School of Human Communication Sciences and Disorders even though my academic background was in psychology. As part of the department, I did a little teaching some years, but just a guest lecturer in the graduate fluency course. As anticipated, my laboratory research was over.

I am not a healthcare professional. In my experience, that was more of a strength than a weakness in this role as dean. Despite my academic appointment formally being in one school, I was not seen as being aligned professionally with that school more than others. I could ask potentially awkward and "naïve" questions of all the schools to make a point and get away with it. My job was not to speak for the different professions—that was the job of each director. My job was to speak for the Faculty to the schools, the university, and the community on issues that transcended individual schools.

I spent much of what would be eleven years as dean focused on breaking down professional school silos and promoting and supporting interprofessional collaboration in education, practice, and research. That activity included presenting (agitating, really) a vision for the Dalhousie to become a national leader in interprofessional education and, as a means to that end, for Dalhousie to construct a special purpose building that would provide a home for interprofessional education. That home would include appropriate and flexible space for interprofessional healthcare simulations, team-based classroom activities and, in a library commons, work spaces in which small groups of students from different professional programs could learn together by working together on projects. Success of the initiative required moving the schools from focusing on traditional siloed think-ing and learning to how to structure their curricula to have their students learn with students from other professional programs. The ultimate goal was to promote teamwork in health care delivery to improve patient care and safety. This goal required my promoting the idea to the senior administration, senior officials in the local health authority, and my colleagues in the Faculty, a challenge because at the time the concepts of collaborative practice and interprofessional education were not generally understood except in a most superficial sense. Most of the planning involved my speaking in one way or another: inspiring, cajoling, arguing, advocating, explaining, pleading, negotiating, mediating, apologizing, using the phone, and participating in and chairing endless meetings, among other things. The building came to be called the Collaborative Health Education Building (CHEB). I felt that all the years I had spent working on my speech had actually paid off. I had become, after 70 years (at that time), a reasonably good communicator. My schoolteachers, my parents, my professors, and many of my former colleagues might not have recognized me. But regardless of how fluent or disfluent my speech was, these meetings and presentations were usually preceded by that same sense of impending loss of control although generally far less so than earlier in my life.

My appointment as dean was extended for an extra year beyond the normal contract end date, and this allowed me to actively participate in the opening of the building in December 2015 by the Honourable Stephen McNeil, Premier of Nova Scotia, and Dr. Richard Florizone, President of Dalhousie. I felt immense satisfaction about the day. During my remarks at the opening, I explained that the theme of the building was reflected in an African proverb that said, "If you want to go fast, go alone; if you want to go far, go together." Premier McNeil's remarks followed mine, and he started by commenting that he was afraid I was going to carry on with the proverb to say, "If you want to go slow, go with government." Lots of warm laughter from everyone. I know that my remarks at the opening, despite my usual self-talk mantras, included some minor blocks and repetitions (bouncing), but that was okay. I really don't think anyone was aware of or cared that I stuttered. And at least anyone who did notice knew from the stuttered speech that it was actually me speaking (with thanks for the line to King George VI, as depicted by Colin Firth in the film, *The King's Speech*).

At least as important as the building were the curricula for the various schools and programs. During my deanship, the concept of collaboration had become embraced by some schools and grudgingly acknowledged by others, and elements of interprofessional education were slowly being embedded in the various curricula (Webster, 2013). As I write this, several years after my retirement, interprofessional education is still alive and strong at Dalhousie. I don't believe that would have happened without the building. Support of the project by the university president, Dr. Tom Traves, approval of the building by the Board of Governors, and partial funding of it by the provincial government sent a clear message to the schools in the Faculty, the rest of the university, and the broader community that interprofessional education and collaborative practice were here to stay. I also don't believe that interprofessional education would still be alive and strong today without the earlier role played by Anne Godden-Webster as interprofessional experience coordinator for the Faculty. She drew upon her previous experience as a clinical educator in speech-language pathology to work patiently and persistently on the front lines with faculty members in the individual schools and with clinical educators in practicum placement sites in the community, encouraging and helping them to develop and implement relevant and meaningful educational and collaborative practice activities to enable students from different programs to work together. Those activities have continued on.

As had been the case at Brock, I had responsibility for reading the names of many of the graduates in my Faculty. The job was a little easier at Dalhousie because students came to the podium one at a time while at Brock they had come came in pairs. As was also the case at Brock, convocation was a time I really did enjoy because of the excitement of the graduates and their families. That did not diminish the apprehension I always experienced beforehand about reading names. However, I did find that, over time, I got better at it; practice really does make perfect (perhaps not perfect, but better). I was always delighted when a member of the audience, often a person who stutters or a family member of someone who stutters, would track me down at the post-ceremony reception to commend me on reading names. From their perspective, I didn't need to be perfect with every name; just the fact that I was a person who stuttered and was on the stage reading names was perfect for them. It was all very gratifying.

As I have reflected on reading names at convocation, it has become clear to me that it is not just the names of people which can be problematic; it is any word in isolation that cannot be changed. I recognized this after I was part of a recent discussion about the difference in meaning, if any, between the words, "burned" and "burnt." This discussion meant frequent use of those two particular words, and it was saying those words in isolation that created difficulties for me. Saying the phrase, for example, "I don't particularly like burnt toast" was not difficult for me, but saying, "I think the word 'burnt' is used more frequently in the UK than in Canada" was difficult because the key word was isolated. This is just like the situation with reading individual names at convocation. Again, avoidance, substitution, and circumlocution are seldom options in these situations. It is that awareness which sets right hemisphere alarms going. In my experience, this is one kind of situation in which using well-practiced fluency skills, including more-effective self-talk strategies, can be a challenge but it is also, for me, where the payoff is greatest.

My retirement as dean in June 2016 took place seven months after the building opening. My office staff organized a wonderful farewell party which of course required lots of circulating and chatting with the guests (not my favourite activity in a large venue) and preparing to make more formal remarks. I was truly touched by the presentations of colleagues and friends from within the university and broader community. In preparing to respond to them, I had prepared my notes with the usual reminders written at the top to use controlled breath and stretch my sounds. My wife, Anne, was in the audience and did an occasional "slow sideways stretching of her arms" to remind me to stretch syllables and slow down. Did I pay attention to her? It was a day like any other.

Retirement Years

My retirement has seen Zoom, Facetime, and Teams, among other platforms, become a ubiquitous part of our culture, and this has meant reliving the apprehension I had around dealing with phone calls in years gone by (and, if I am being honest, I still have). Before a group call or meeting on Zoom starts, I have that same sense of impending loss of control (and not an unrealistic sense given several negative speech experiences I have had on Zoom). During the Zoom call, I have constant apprehension about how and when to start speaking, and indeed where to look. The familiar social cues are not there, and unlike in face-to-face meetings, I can see myself on the screen. I find that distracting and, because it makes me motivated to withdraw, it is right hemisphere activating. I recognize that much of the problem is an unfamiliar social script for which I need more experience. One-on-one Zoom or Facetime calls are better than group meetings for me, even when the group may have just three or four participants. So, dealing with this has become one of my current speech projects. Another project stems from my having less phone use in my current retired life, and I am finding more difficulty in using the phone. It is hard work and sometimes—this is confession time—I just give in to avoidance and ask Anne to phone for me.

I discussed earlier the challenge I experienced as a new department chair participating in round-table introductions at meetings or other gatherings. This challenge continues today, and not just on Zoom. In my exercise class with 30-40 participants, many of whom I know reasonably well, we routinely go around the room saying our first names just to remind one another who is who. I've been surprised to find that as this process starts, that old sense of impending loss of control gets fired up, I stop listening, and prepare to say "Will" when my turn comes. Over my several years in the class, I have never blocked or hesitated or prolonged in saying "Will," but still the anxiety about the possibility of stuttering continues. What has changed is that I now have the means of (usually) countering that anxiety and controlling my speech. But it does take a moment of conscious planning. Old fears die hard.

In the Introduction, I commented on the experiences of Dr. Charles Van Riper, a well-known speech-language pathologist of the last century, who lamented about his stuttering getting worse with age. I am finding the same. Perhaps I am just getting out of practice in speaking, and the principle of "use it or lose it" may apply. These days, I am not pushed much; in retirement there are simply fewer opportunities to be pushed into speaking situations. My formal leadership roles have been limited so far to participating on the boards of a couple of not-for-profit organizations. There are fewer social and professional expectations of me, and there are many fewer things that I feel I should be doing (apart from writing this book). For me, improved fluency over the years has required the **conscious application of**

skills. Following from the discussion at the end of chapter 7, I suspect that if those skills aren't used consistently, the neuronal links proposed by Dr. Hebb may weaken and old habits return. But, of course, the increased stuttering with age may also simply reflect the putative changes in the brain that come with age. It is beyond the scope of this book and well beyond my expertise to speculate on what those changes might be and how they might impact stuttering. It is my hope—indeed my dream—that a reader of this book, perhaps a graduate student or faculty member in speech science or neuroscience, might become interested in and motivated to carry out systematic research into this question of aging and stuttering and, indeed, into other aspects of what the Two-Factor Model has to say about stuttering and its management at all ages.

CHAPTER 9

What has the Brain Taught Me?

S tuttering is hard work! Managing stuttering is also hard work! For some, stuttering therapy with a focus on stutter-free speech may be the chosen route for managing speech and communication; for others, stuttering therapy with a focus on stuttering modification, or voluntary stuttering, or reducing fear and apprehension, or enhancing self-esteem may be the chosen route; for others, participating in a self-help group may be the chosen route; and for still others, courageously forging ahead, ever hopeful, may be the chosen (or imposed by circumstance) route. Each route is hard, requires focus, perseverance, patience, flexibility, and resilience.

This concluding chapter pulls together some of what I think I have learned about stuttering during the first 80 years of my life. I want to put that discussion into the context of the Two-Factor Interference Model of stuttering, which is included here again as figure 5. I'm going to start by discussing this model or theory in a slightly different way than I did earlier, and then move on to strategies for managing stuttering that I believe flow from the theory and from my personal experiences.

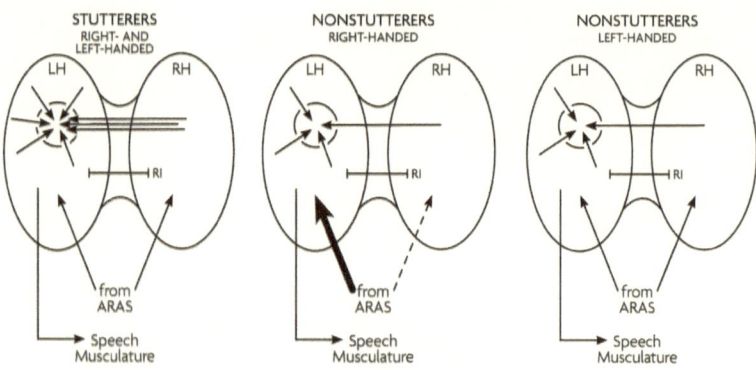

Figure 5. Two-factor Interference Model of Stuttering. LEFT DIAGRAM: Right-
and left-handed stutterers; MIDDLE DIAGRAM: Right-handed non-stutterers;
RIGHT DIAGRAM: Left-handed non-stutterers. (LH=left hemisphere; RH=right
hemisphere; RI=reciprocal inhibition; ARAS=ascending reticular activating system)

If one, as a person who stutters, is to facilitate relatively stutter-free
speech, the goal under the Two-Factor Interference Model is to **maximize
left** hemisphere (LH) supplementary motor area (SMA) activity and to
minimize right hemisphere (RH) activity. Drawing upon the research
findings in earlier chapters and upon some speculation on my part, the key
elements of the Model entail the following:

- The SMA of the LH is involved in the planning, organization, and
  initiation of speech motor movements. To do this, the SMA must
  receive and process kinesthetic information from the speech musculature and integrate that kinesthetic information with other motor
  planning and initiation processes. When the SMA has access to
  kinesthetic feedback and when the SMA is working efficiently with
  minimal interference, the result can be coordinated motor movements and stutter-free speech.

- The LH SMA is vulnerable to interference from other brain activity,
  especially that occurring in the RH. That vulnerability impacts on
  the efficiency of the SMA in processing kinesthetic feedback and in
  organizing speech movements. Overactivity of the RH may overflow
  to the LH SMA through the corpus callosum.

- RH activity may increase when one (stutterer or non-stutterer) experiences negative emotions like fear and apprehension or, more generally, when one is motivated to withdraw from a situation.
- Because people who stutter lack a LH activation bias, their RH may become more readily activated than is the case for people who do not stutter.
- The level of RH activity can also increase due to reduced reciprocal inhibition acting on the RH when LH activity is low. LH activity will be low when fluency skills are not being used and attention is not being focused on the feel (kinesthesis) of controlled speech movements.
- When LH activity is low, the SMA is inefficient in integrating kinesthetic information into motor planning and initiation processes, resulting in dis-coordinated muscle movements that are manifest as stuttering.
- LH activity can increase (increasing the efficiency with which kinesthetic information can be processed) when RH activity decreases. This can occur when negative emotions to withdraw from a situation are brought under control (through, for example, more-effective self-talk, progressive relaxation exercises).
- LH activity can increase when the emotions being experienced are positive and motivate one to enter and engage in a situation.
- LH activity can increase (along with efficiency with which kinesthetic information can be processed) with intentional focusing of attention on the feel and organization of speech movements.
- The bottom line: When LH activity is relatively high and RH activity is relatively low, the LH SMA is able to work more efficiently in planning, organizing, and initiating speech movements that support relatively fluent speech.

Reflection Note to the Reader

Before reading further, spend a few minutes thinking about what the elements of the Two Factor Theory just outlined might suggest about strategies for managing speech. Be as specific as you can. What can a person who stutters actually do (at least in principle) to impact their

---

stuttering? Don't hesitate to bring in relevant more-effective self-talk (see the Appendix Tables for specific examples). Referring to the model, what is the basis for your suggestions? Write down some of your ideas and compare them against what follows.

When you are ready to continue, the following are some suggestions that I might make. After the first two, they are in no particular order.

- Learn to use speech motor movements controlled by the left hemisphere that will facilitate stutter-free speech. This is most effectively done by taking advantage of an individual or group treatment program offered in-person or virtually by a trained speech-language pathologist. **Managing stuttering ultimately requires managing speech motor movements**. The skills may include proper breathing, controlled speech rate, stretched sounds, having smooth vocalization onsets, linking sounds, and using deliberate and possibly exaggerated speech movements.

- Accept that fear and its brother, avoidance, are **not** your friends. **Don't avoid speaking situations**; don't procrastinate; and don't hold back on matters that require speaking. Avoidance generates fears and anxieties and allows them to percolate and fester, resulting in increased right hemisphere activity.

- Practice using **more-effective self-talk** with supportive thoughts and actions to control fears. As apprehension, fear, or motivation to withdraw from a speaking situation is reduced, right hemisphere activation and its potential to interfere with speech motor control may be reduced.

- **Be proactive** and find opportunities to speak. **Don't hold back—** make this your mantra! Take the initiative to introduce yourself, to go first with giving a short report to your group, to thank someone for a favour, to offer a toast at a wedding, to ask for needed directions, to make a phone call to make an appointment, and the list goes on. Being proactive and prepared brings out positive emotions related going into a situation rather withdrawing from a situation.

- Respond positively to being **pushed** by family, friends, employers, etc. into situations that require speaking. Or better still, don't wait to be pushed: **reach out** and **volunteer**. And when you volunteer, use more effective self-talk to generate positive motivations, not dread, about approaching the situation. Make the commitments well ahead if you can. And use the time to plan how you can be successful, however you want to define success. Think about the self-talk you may want to use and write it down. Having planned what you want to say and how you are going to say it will facilitate left hemisphere activation at the time of speaking and, through addressing fear in the preparation, will decrease right hemisphere activation.

- And if you are not sure what to say or how to say it in some situation and are feeling uneasy or uncomfortable, consider whether you need some advice and help on **polishing your social skills** in that particular area. The effect of being uncomfortable in that situation is that you will want to withdraw from it, and that is associated with right hemisphere activation and interference.

- Cultivate **active listening** skills with good **eye contact**. Active listening will help you ignore that sense of impending loss of control and help you focus on what you want to say, not just how you want to say it. Drawing yourself into a speaking situation, like a conversation, is an example of generating **approach** that supports LH activity. Maintaining eye contact conveys to others and confers on the speaker self-confidence and self-worth.

- If you have had a disappointing situation, even a disappointing speech day, as we all do, remember the adage about being thrown from a horse—pick yourself up, re-mount, and ride. Doing so prevents what is called the "**incubation of anxiety**" effect—anxiety that increases with just the passage of time.

- Take opportunities to **disclose** openly and proudly that you are a person who stutters. There is **no shame** in it. Be proud of your efforts to learn about and deal with stuttering and share with others something about what you have learned or are currently learning and putting into practice. If the fact of your stuttering remains a secret, any speech hesitation or repetition or blockage will be a disclosure of that secret, and trying to maintain secrecy will contribute to apprehension and consequently to right hemisphere activation. Openness (a form of approach motivation) decreases right hemisphere activation and so, through reduced reciprocal inhibition on the left hemisphere, left hemisphere SMA activity will increase which in turn facilitates or supports use of speech fluency skills. Anticipate questions and comments from others by developing brief (20-30 second) "elevator pitch" initial answers so you don't feel rushed or flustered. (Remember that an answer can start with, "I don't know but...")

- Learn how to apply **progressive relaxation** or similar techniques so you have a means of responding to tension you experience in speaking situations. When you engage in progressive relaxation, you can reduce right hemisphere activity which in turn enhances the operation of the left hemisphere SMA. Practicing progressive relaxation before a speaking event can distract from worry and give a real sense of control.

- Periodically during the day engage in a couple of minutes of **slow and exaggerated speaking** to "loosen up" the system and get the kinesthetic feedback flowing.

- **Join** and become **an active participant** in organizations such as the Canadian Stuttering Association, the National Stuttering Association (in the United States), or the British Stammering Association, as well as a self-help group in your community. As you gain more control over your speech, consider joining a community public speaking group like Toastmasters˙. Take advantage of these opportunities to learn more about stuttering, to meet others who stutter, to practice common social scripts while maintaining eye contact, and especially to have fun!

- **Above all else, be kind to yourself and be self-forgiving!**

When I was working with the groups of people who stutter, I would encourage everyone to read, think about, and discuss in the group a short piece written many years ago by Dr. J. David Williams, a well-known and respected speech-language pathologist specializing in stuttering treatment. It is reprinted below and very much captures how I have come to feel about what constitutes success for someone who stutters. In 1988, while he was still alive and a professor emeritus at Northern Illinois University, Professor Williams gave Marie Poulos and me permission to include the piece in our *Facilitating Fluency* manual, and it is reprinted here. (I have not changed the use of gendered pronouns and would ask the reader to make the appropriate substitutions).

* * * * * * * *

The Successful Stutterer
by J. David Williams

A "successful stutterer," as defined here, does not mean an "ex-stutterer" who has completely recovered from his stuttering problem and will never again have any of the speech behaviors nor any of the attitudes and feelings that made up his stuttering problem. It does mean a stutterer who is working his way toward recovery, who is making significant progress and who continues to do everything he can to maximize that progress. What does he think, and do? In my opinion, the successful stutterer:

- Has, to whatever degree he finds necessary, learned to modify his everyday speaking behavior in such a way as to minimize the occurrence of stuttering blocks, and/or has learned to modify the manner in which he stutters when blocks do occur. To do either, he has selected from a variety of possible modification techniques one or more that he is willing and able to use in a consistent manner so that he gains a feeling of fairly predictable control over his stuttering.

- Knows that whatever the basic nature of stuttering, the most disruptive aspect of the problem is fear of stuttering and his consequent and generally ineffective efforts to deny, conceal, and avoid its occurrence. Knows that fear disrupts both rational thinking and voluntary control of motor behaviour (including speech), and that if, at a given moment, his fear reaches a certain intensity, it is literally impossible for him to successfully carry out any of the voluntary modification techniques he has learned.

- Has learned to keep his fear of stuttering within manageable limits. Does not give way to blind panic at the approach of a feared speaking situation. Realizes he cannot wish away his old, well-conditioned fear responses, but has learned how to override the fear and go ahead and talk. On the relatively few occasions that his anxiety-tensions do get out of hand in a speaking situation, he does not

157

regard it as a disaster; rather, he chalks it up to experience and tries to keep his feelings under better control next time.

- Realizes that what he **does** about his stuttering problem is more important than what he **says** and **thinks** about it. Knows that the feelings and behaviors of stuttering are modified and brought under control more by action (voluntary experimenting with and practicing self-changes in real life situations) than by **insight** (gaining intellectual knowledge of the problem and one's reactions to it), but that action **plus** insight is best of all.

- Knows that real and permanent change in feelings and behaviors does not happen easily, quickly, or automatically. The stuttering problem took a long time to develop and will not vanish overnight. Realizes that improvement will come in direct proportion to amount of active, sustained, daily effort he expends. Knows that many small successes cumulate to produce a more permanent change than does one spectacular event. Is motivated for long range self-monitoring and is not discouraged by the temporary setbacks, whether internally or externally caused, that inevitably occur. Does not depend on external sources of motivation but is self-motivated by the feeling of achievement and progress derived from personal effort.

- Has a basic self-respect, a feeling of self-worth. Does not allow the stuttering problem to overwhelm and destroy him. Has a sense of perspective: tries to keep a realistic view of the ways in which stuttering really is a handicap and more numerous ways in which it is not. Tries to develop and capitalize on all his personal assets. Identifies with people in general, does not fear them—has more of an "approach" than "avoidance" attitude toward others. Knows that all people have common denominators of fears and insecurities from many causes. Minimizes debilitating self-pity and tries to maximize a positive-outward looking attitude. Has a positive, non-self-deprecating sense of humor. **Enjoys life.**

> **"Whatever you can do, or dream you can do, begin it.**
> **Boldness has genius, power, and magic in it."**
> Johann Wolfgang Von Goethe (1749-1832).

CONCLUDING COMMENTS

I would like to thank you, the reader, for accompanying me on this journey of my personal and professional relationship with stuttering. The personal relationship has been lifelong; the professional relationship has been shorter and began as a result of the curious experiences I described in chapters 3 and 4 that seemed to link a marked improvement in my speech fluency to being on a low carbohydrate weight-loss diet. The subsequent discussions and speculations with my friend on the bus to the Oxford conference provided an impetus for me to explore the brain mechanisms underlying stuttering. I never did get back to the question about whether there was a real effect of diet to be studied, and if so, what might underlie it neurologically or neurochemically. I retain an open mind about that issue but accept that at my age and stage I will not now be the one investigating it.

Part II, encompassing chapters 4-7, was entitled, "Time to set the world on fire." That title was based on the advice I had received from Dr. Donald Hebb of McGill University when I was a graduate student at Cornell. As I recounted in chapter 3, he advised me to finish my graduate training as soon as possible and then, once I was appointed to a university faculty position, it was "time to set the world on fire." Seventy-five years ago, when Dr. Hebb published his book, *The Organization of Behavior,* he really did set on fire the worlds of neuroscience and psychology, and the embers are still glowing today. My research has certainly **not** "set the world on fire," but I would like to think that it has cast some new and useful light on how to think about stuttering and its management. It is my hope that by my having shared this journey, the reader will have an appreciation of both the complexity of stuttering, and also the simplicity of the Two-Factor Interference Model as a means for understanding stuttering. My hope is that the Model and its implications will be as useful to you, the reader, as it has been to me. Stuttering can be managed although I don't suggest it is easy. But it is worth the effort.

I have had the privilege of being in a position through my career to have been engaged in personally meaningful research and teaching activities, to have worked closely with people who stutter, and to have held a number of university leadership positions that have helped my stuttering by requiring me to speak in so many different contexts. Now I look back over my life and am quite astonished that I would have accepted and welcomed the positions I have held. When I was a young person who struggled with speaking, I would never have imagined that my life would have unfolded in this way. However, at this stage of my life, I cannot imagine my life not having unfolded in much the way it has. It is my hope that this story, which began in early childhood and continues until today, 80 years later, can be a source of some inspiration, encouragement, and empowerment for people who stutter to step up to the plate and become the leaders that this world needs. As Dr. Seuss famously said:

"Why fit in when you were born to stand out?"

REFERENCES

Ahern, G.L., & Schwartz, G.E. (1985). Differential lateralization for positive and negative emotion in the human brain: EEG spectral analysis. *Neuropsychologia, 23*, 745-755.

Albanese, E., Merlo, A., Albanese, A., & Gomez, E. (1989). Anterior speech region: Asymmetry and weight-surface correlation. *Archives of Neurology, 46*, 307-310.

Alm, P.A. (2004). Stuttering and the basal ganglia circuits: a critical review of possible relations. *Journal of Communication Disorders, 37*, 325-369.

Andrews, G., Craig, A., Feyer, A.-M., Hoddinott, S., Howie, P., and Neilson, M. (1983). Stuttering: a review of research findings and theories circa 1982. *Journal of Speech and Hearing Disorders, 48*, 226-246.

Andrews, G., & Harris, M.M. (1964). The syndrome of stuttering. *Clinics in Developmental Medicine, No. 17.* London: Spastics Society Medical Education and Information Unit/Heinemann.

Andrews, G., Quinn, P.T., & Sorby, W.A. (1972). Stuttering: an investigation into cerebral dominance for speech. *Journal of Neurology, Neurosurgery and Psychiatry, 35*, 414-418.

Annett, M. (1978). *A single gene explanation of right and left handedness and brainedness.* Coventry: Lanchester Polytechnic.

Bair, J.H. (1901). Development of voluntary control. *Psychological Review, 8*, 474-510.

Blood, G. W. (1985). Laterality differences in child stutterers: Heterogeneity, severity levels, and statistical treatments. *Journal of Speech and Hearing Disorders, 50*, 66-72.

Bloodstein, O. (1981). *A handbook on stuttering* (3rd ed.), Chicago, IL: National Easter Seal Society.

Boberg, E. (1993). *Neuropsychology of stuttering*. Edmonton: University of Alberta Press.

Boberg, E., & Kully, D. (1985). *A comprehensive stuttering program*. San Diego, CA: College-Hill Press.

Boberg, E. & Webster, W.G. (1990) Stuttering: Current status of theory and therapy. *Canadian Family Physician, 36*, 1156-1160.

Boberg, E., Yeudall, L.T., Schopflocher, D., & Bo-Lassen, P. (1983). The effect of an intensive behavioral program on the distribution of EEG alpha power in stutterers during the processing of verbal and visuospatial information. *Journal of Fluency Disorders, 8*, 245-263.

Box, G.E.P. (1976). Science and statistics. *Journal of the American Statistical Association, 71*, 791-799.

Bradshaw, J.L., & Nettleton, N.C. (1983). *Human cerebral asymmetry*. Englewood Cliffs: Prentice-Hall.

Brady, J.P. & Berson, J. (1975). Stuttering: dichotic listening, and cerebral dominance. *Archives of General Psychiatry, 32*, 1449-1452.

Braun, A.R., Varga, M., Stager, S., Schulz, G., Selbie, S., Maisog, J.M., Carson, R.E. & Ludlow, C.C. (1997). Atypical lateralization of hemispheral activity in development stuttering: An H_2 ^{15}O positron emission tomography study. In W. Hulstijn, H.F.M. Peters, & P.H.H.M. van Lieshout (Eds.), *Speech production: Motor control, brain research and fluency disorders* (pp. 279-292). Amsterdam: Elsevier.

Brinkman, C. (1984). Supplementary motor area of the monkey's cerebral cortex: Short- and long-term deficits after unilateral ablation and the effects of subsequent callosal section. *Journal of Neuroscience, 4*, 918-929.

Brito, G.N.O. & Webster, W.G. (1979). Electrophysiological indicant of asymmetric hemispheric involvement in discrimination performance by cat. *Brain Research, 175*, 150-154.

Bryden, M.P. (1978). Strategy effects in the assessment of hemispheric asymmetries. In G. Underwood (Ed.), *Strategies of information processing*. New York: Academic Press.

Bryden, M.P. (1982). *Laterality: Functional asymmetry in the intact brain*. New York: Academic Press.

Bryden, M.P., & Mondor, T.A. (1991). Attentional factors in visual field asymmetries. *Canadian Journal of Psychology, 45*, 427-447.

Cain, S. (2013*). Quiet: The power of introverts in a world that can't stop talking*. New York: Random House (Crown).

Caruso, A. J., Abbs, J.H., & Gracco, V.L. (1988). Kinematic analysis of multiple movement coordination during speech in stutterers. *Brain, 111*, 439-455).

Cohen, G. (1982). Theoretical interpretations. In J.G. Beaumont (Ed.), *Divided visual field studies of cerebral organization*. New York; Academic Press.

Coren, S. (1992). *The left-hander syndrome: The causes and consequences of left-handedness*. Free Press.

Curry, F.K.W., & Gregory, H.H. (1969). The performance of stutterers on dichotic listening tasks thought to reflect verbal dominance. *Journal of Speech and Hearing Research, 12*, 73-82.

Davidson, R.J. (1984). Hemispheric asymmetry and emotion. In K.R. Scherer & P. Ekman (Eds.), *Approaches to emotion*. Hillsdale, NJ: Erlbaum.

Davidson, R.J., Fox, N.A. (1981). Asymmetrical brain activity discriminates between positive versus negative affective stimuli in ten-month-old infants. *Science, 218*, 1235-1237.

De Nil, L.F., Kroll, R.M., Kapur, S., & Houle, S. (2000). A positron emission tomography study of silent and oral single word reading in stuttering and nonstuttering adults. *Journal of Speech, Language, and Hearing Research, 43*, 1038-1053.

Denkla, M.B. (1983). Development of speed in repetitive and successive finger-movements in normal children. *Developmental Medicine and Child Neurology, 15*, 635-645.

Forster, D.C. (1996). *Speech-motor control and interhemispheric relations in recovered and persistent stuttering.* PhD dissertation, Carleton University, Ottawa, Ontario, Canada.

Forster, D.C. & Webster, W.G. (1991). Concurrent task interference in stutterers: Dissociating hemispheric specialization and activation. *The Canadian Journal of Psychology, 45*, 321-335.

Forster, D.C., & Webster, W.G. (2001). Speech-motor control and interhemispheric relations in recovered and persistent stuttering. *Developmental Neuropsychology, 19*, 125-145.

Foundas, A.L., Leonard, C.M., & Heilman, K.M. (1995). Morphologic cerebral asymmetries and handedness. *Archives of Neurology, 52*, 501-508.

Fox. N.A., & Davidson, R.J. (1988). Patterns of brain electrical activity during facial signs of emotion in 10-month-old infants. *Developmental Psychology, 24*, 130-136.

Fox, P.T., Ingham, R.J., Ingham, J.C., Hirsch, T., Downs, J.H., Martin, C., Jerabek, P., Glass, R., & Lancaster, J.L. (1996). A PET study of the neural systems of stuttering. *Nature, 382*, 158-162.

Galaburda, A.M., LeMay, M., Kemper, T.L., & Geschwind, N. (1978). Right-left asymmetries in the brain. *Science, 199*, 852-856.

Gazzaniga, M.S. (1983). Right hemisphere language following brain bisection. *American Psychologist, 38*, 525-537.

Geschwind, N., & Levitsky, W. (1968). Human brain: Left-right asymmetries in temporal speech region. *Science, 161*, 186-187.

Goldberg, G. (1985). Supplementary motor area structure and function: Review and hypotheses. *The Behavioral and Brain Sciences, 8*, 567-616.

Goodale, M.A. (1988). Hemispheric differences in motor control. *Behavioural Brain Research, 30*, 203-214.

Halsband, U., Matsuzaka, Y., & Tanji, J. (1994). Neuronal activity in the primate supplementary, pre-supplementary and premotor cortex during externally and internally instructed sequential movements. *Neuroscience Research, 20,* 149-155.

Hayes, T.L., & Lewis, D.A. (1985). Anatomical specialization of the anterior motor speech area: Hemispheric differences in magnopyramidal neurons. *Brain and Language, 49,* 289-308.

Hebb, D.O. (1949). *The organization of behavior.* New York: John Wiley & Sons.

Howie, P.M. (1981). Concordance for stuttering in monozygotic and dizygotic twin pairs. *Journal of Speech and Hearing Research, 24,* 317-321.

Ikeda, A., Luders, H.O., Shibasaki, H., Collura, T.F., Burgess, R.C, Morris, H.H., & Hamano, T. (1995). Movement-related potentials associated with bilateral simultaneous and unilateral movements recorded from human supplementary motor area. *Electroencephalography and Clinical Neurophysiology, 95,* 323-334.

Ingham, R.J. (2004). Emerging controversies, findings, and direction in neuroimaging and developmental stuttering: On avoiding petard hoisting in Athens, Georgia. In A. Bothe (Ed.), *Evidenced-Based Practice in Stuttering* (pp. 27-63). New York: Lawrence Erlbaum Associates.

Ingham, R.J., Fox, P.T., Ingham, J.C. (1997). A $H_2^{15}O$ positron emission tomography (PET) study on adults who stutter: Findings and implications. In W. Hulstijn, H.F.M., & P.H.H.M. van Lieshout (Eds.), *Speech production: Motor control, brain research and fluency disorders* (pp. 293-305). Amsterdam: Elsevier.

Ingham, R.J., Fox, P.T., Ingham, J.C., & Zamarripa, F. (2000). Is overt stuttered speech a prerequisite for the neural activations associated with chronic developmental stuttering? *Brain and Language, 75,* 163-194.

Ingham, R.J., Ingham, J.C., Euler, H.A., & Neumann, K. (2018). Stuttering treatment and brain research in adults: A still unfolding relationship. *Journal of Fluency Disorders, 55,* 106-119.

James, W. (1890). *Principles of Psychology.* New York: Henry Holt.

Johannsen, H.S., & Victor, C. (1986). Visual information processing in the left and right hemispheres during unilateral tachistoscopic stimulation of stutterers. *Journal of Fluency Disorders, 11*, 285-291.

Kidd, K.K. (1984). Stuttering as a genetic disorder. In R.F. Curlee & W.H. Perkins (Eds.), *The nature and treatment of stuttering: New directions*. San Diego, CA: College-Hill Press, pp. 149-169.

Kimble, G. A., & Perlmuter, L. C. (1970). The problem of volition. *Psychological Review, 77*(5), 361–384.

Kimura, D. (1982). Left-hemisphere control of oral and brachial movements and their relation to communication. *Philosophical transactions of the Royal Society of London, B298*, 135-149.

Kimura, D. (1993). *Neuromotor mechanisms in human communication*. Oxford University Press.

Kinsbourne, M. (1974). Lateral interactions in the brain. In M. Kinsbourne & W. L. Smith (Eds.), *Hemispheric disconnection and cerebral function* (pp. 239–259). Charles C Thomas.

Kinsbourne, M., & McMurray, J. (1975). The effect of cerebral dominance on time sharing between speaking and tapping by preschool children. *Child Development, 46*, 240-242.

Kushner, H.I. (2011). Retraining left-handers and the aetiology of stuttering: The rise and fall of an intriguing theory. *Laterality, 17*, 673-693.

Lang, W., Obrig, H., Lindinger, G., Cheyne, D., & Deecke, L. (1990). Supplementary motor area activation while tapping bimanually different rhythms in musicians. *Experimental Brain Research, 79*, 504-514.

Lomas, J., & Kimura, D. (1976). Interhemispheric interaction between speaking and sequential manual activity. *Neuropsychologia, 14*, 23-33.

Luessenhop, A.J., Boggs, J.S., Lorowit, L.J., & Walle, E.L. (1973). Cerebral dominance in stutterers determined by Wada testing. *Neurology, 23*, 1190-1192.

Martin, D. & Webster, W.G. (1974). Paw preference shifts in the rat following forced practice. *Physiology and Behavior, 13*, 745-748.

Mateer, C.A. (1983). Motor and perceptual functions of the left hemisphere and their interaction. In S. Segalowitz (Ed.), *Language functions and brain organization* (pp. 145-170). New York: Academic Press.

McGilchrist, I. (2010). Reciprocal organization of the cerebral hemispheres. *Dialogues in Clinical Neuroscience, 12*(4), 503-513.

Milner, B., Branch, D., & Rasmussen, T. (1966). Evidence for bilateral speech representation in some non-right-handers. *Transactions of the American Neurological Association, 91,* 306-308.

Mondor, T.A. & Bryden, M.P. (1991). The influence of attention on the dichotic REA. *Neuropsychologia, 29* (12), 1179-1190.

Mondor, T.A., & Bryden, M.P. (1992). On the relation between visual spatial attention and visual field asymmetries. *The Quarterly Journal of Experimental Psychology, 44,* 529-555.

Moore, W.H. (1976). Bilateral tachistoscopic word perception of stutterers and normal subjects. *Brain and Language, 3,* 434-442.

Moore, W.H. (1986). Hemispheric alpha asymmetries of stutterers and nonstutterers for the recall and recognition of words and connected reading passages: Some relationships to severity of stuttering. *Journal of Fluency Disorders, 11,* 71-89.

Moore, W.H. (1993). Hemispheric processing research. In E. Boberg (Ed.), *Neuropsychology of stuttering* (pp. 39-72). Edmonton: University of Alberta Press.

Moore, W.H., & Haynes, W.O. (1980). Alpha hemispheric asymmetry and stuttering: Some support for a segmentation dysfunction hypothesis. *Journal of Speech and Hearing Research, 23,* 229-247.

Mountcasle, V.B. (1962). *Interhemispheric relations and cerebral dominance.* Baltimore: Johns Hopkins Press.

Mushiake, H., Inase, M., & Tanji, J. (1990). Selective coding of motor sequence in supplementary motor area of the monkey cerebral cortex. *Experimental Brain Research, 82,* 208-210.

Ojemann, G.A. (1983). Brain organization for language from the perspective of electrical stimulation mapping. *The Behavioral and Brain Sciences, 2,* 189-230.

Orton, S.T. (1928). A physiological theory of reading disability and stuttering in children. *New England Journal of Medicine, 199,* 1046-1052.

Passingham, R.E., Chen, Y.C., & Thaler, D. (1989). Supplementary motor cortex and self-initiated movements. In M. Ito (Ed.), *Neural programing (Taniguchi Symposia on brain sciences No. 12)* (pp. 13-24). Basal: S. Karger.

Penfield, W., & Welch, K. (1949). The supplementary motor area in the cerebral cortex of man. *Transactions of the American Neurological Association, 74,* 79-84.

Perecman, E. (Ed.). (1983). *Cognitive Processing in the right hemisphere.* New York: Academic Press.

Perkins, W.H. (1983). The problem of definition. *Journal of Speech and Hearing Disorders, 48,* 246-249.

Perkins, W.H. (1985). Horizons and beyond: Confessions of a carpenter. *Seminars in Speech and Language, 6,* 233-244.

Peters, M. (1980). Why the preferred hand taps more quickly than the non-preferred hand: Three experiments on handedness. *Canadian Journal of Psychology, 34,* 62-71.

Peters, M. (1987). A nontrivial motor performance difference between right-handers and left-handers: Attention as an intervening variable in the expression of handedness. *Canadian Journal of Psychology, 41,* 91-99.

Poulos, M., & Webster, W.G. (1991). Family history as a basis for subgrouping people who stutter. *Journal of Speech and Hearing Research, 34,* 5-10.

Preilowski, B. (1972). Possible contribution of the anterior forebrain commissures to bilateral motor coordination. *Neuropsychologia, 10,* 267-277.

Rastatter, M.P., & Dell, C.W. (1987). Reaction times of moderate and severe stutterers to monaural verbal stimuli: Some implications for neurolinguistic organization. *Journal of Speech and Hearing Research,* *30*, 21-27.

Riley, G.D., Wu, J.C., & Maguire, G. (1997). PET scan evidence of parallel cerebral systems related to treatment effects. In W. Hulstijn, H.F.M. Peters, & P.H.H.M. van Lieshout (Eds.), *Speech production: Motor control, brain research and fluency disorders* (pp. 321-339. Amsterdam: Elsevier.

Roland, P.E. (1984a). Organization of motor control by the normal human brain. *Human Neurobiology, 2*, 205-216.

Roland, P.E. (1984b). Metabolic measurements of the working frontal cortex in man. *Trends in Neuroscience, 7*, 430-435.

Roland, P.E. (1985). Cortical organization of voluntary behavior in man. *Human Neurobiology, 4*, 155-167.

Roland, P.E., Larsen, B., Lassen, N.A., & Skinhoj, E. (1980). Supplementary motor area and other cortical areas in organization of voluntary movements in man. *Journal of Neurophysiology, 43*, 118-136.

Rosenfield, D.B., & Goodglass, H. (1980). Dichotic testing of cerebral dominance in stutterers. *Brain and Language, 11*, 170-180.

Rouiller, E.M., Babalian, A., Kazennikov, O., Moret, V., Yu, X.-H., & Wiesendanger, M. (1994). Transcallosal connections of the distal forelimb representations of the primary and supplementary motor cortical areas in macaque monkeys. *Experimental Brain Research, 102*, 227-243.

Searleman, A. (1977). A review of right hemisphere linguistic capabilities. *Psychological Bulletin, 84*, 503-528.

Simonetta, M., Clanet, M., & Roscol, O. (1991). Bereitschaftspotential in a simple movement or in a motor sequence starting with the same simple movement. *Electroencephalography and clinical Neurophysiology, 81*, 129-134l

Sperry, R.W. (1974). Lateral specialization in the surgically separated hemispheres. In F.O. Schmitt & F.G. Worden (Eds.), *The neurosciences: Third study program* (pp. 5-20). Cambridge, Mass.: MIT Press.

Tanji, J. (1994). The supplementary motor area in the cerebral cortex. *Neuroscience Research, 19*, 251-268.

Tanji, J., & Shima, K. (1994). Role for supplementary motor area cells in planning several movements ahead. *Nature, 371*, 413-416.

Todor, J.I., & Kyrie, P.M. (1980). Hand differences in the rate and variability of rapid tapping. *Journal of Motor Behavior, 12*, 57-62.

Travis, L.E. (1931). *Speech pathology*. New York: Appleton.

Travis, L.E. (1978). The cerebral dominance theory of stuttering: 1931-1978. *Journal of Speech and Hearing Disorders, 43*, 278-281.

Treisman, A.M. (1965). The effects of redundancy and familiarity on translating and repeating back a foreign and a native language. *British Journal of Psychology, 56*, 369-379.

Van Riper, C. (1934). A new test of laterality. *Journal of Experimental Psychology, 17*, 305-313.

Warren, J.M., & Akert, K. (Eds.). (1964). *The frontal granular cortex and behavior*. McGraw-Hill.

Warren, J.M., Cornwell, P.R., Webster, W.G., & Pubols, B.H. (1972). Unilateral cortical lesions and paw preferences in cats. *Journal of Comparative and Physiological Psychology, 81*, 410-422.

Webster, E.C. (Au.), Webster, W.G. (Ed.), Webster, D.E.G. (Ed.). (2023). *Origins of Professional Psychology in Canada (1925-1965): Reflections of a pioneer*. Winnipeg: Friesen Press.

Webster, R.L. (1980). Evolution of a target-based behavioral therapy for stuttering. *Journal of Fluency Disorders, 5*, 303-320.

Webster, R.L., & Stoeckel, C.M. (1984). *Precision fluency shaping program: Speech reconstruction for stutterers*. Roanoke, VA.: Communications Development Corp.

Webster, W.G. (1972). Functional asymmetry between the cerebral hemispheres of the cat. *Neuropsychologia, 10*: 75-87.

Webster, W.G. (1973). Assumptions, conceptualizations, and the search for the functions of the brain. *Physiological Psychology, 1*, 346-350. [Reprinted as Conceptualizations of brain function, in M. Marx & F.A. Goodson (Eds.), *Theories of Contemporary Psychology*, 2nd edition (pp. 458-468). New York: Macmillan, 1976.

Webster, W.G. (1975). *Principles of Research Methodology in Physiological Psychology.* New York: Harper & Row.

Webster, W.G. (1977). Territoriality and the evolution of brain asymmetry. In S.J. Dimond & D.A. Blizard (Eds.), *Evolution and lateralization of the brain* (pp. 213-221). New York: New York Academy of Sciences. (Published as Volume 299 of the *Annals of the New York Academy of Sciences.*) (Translated and reprinted in 1982 as La territorialidad y la evolucion de la asimetria cerebral. In J.E. Ortega (Ed.), *Lecturas Sobre Comportamiento Animal* (pp. 205-219). Madrid: Siglo XXI de Espana Editores, S.A.)

Webster, W.G. (1985). Neuropsychological models of stuttering -- I. Representation of sequential response mechanisms. *Neuropsychologia, 23*, 263-267.

Webster, W.G. (1986a). Response sequence organization and reproduction by stutterers. *Neuropsychologia, 24*, 813-821.

Webster, W.G. (1986b). Neuropsychological models of stuttering -- II. Interhemispheric interference. *Neuropsychologia, 24*, 737-741.

Webster, W.G. (1987). Rapid letter transcription performance by stutterers. *Neuropsychologia, 25*, 845-847.

Webster, W.G. (1988). Neural mechanisms underlying stuttering: Evidence from bimanual handwriting. *Brain and Language, 33*, 226-244.

Webster, W.G. (1989a). Sequence initiation by stutterers under conditions of response competition. *Brain and Language, 36*, 286-300.

Webster, W.G. (1989b). Sequence reproduction deficits in stutterers tested under nonspeeded response conditions. *Journal of Fluency Disorders, 14*, 79-86.

Webster, W.G. (1990a). Evidence in bimanual finger tapping of an attentional component to stuttering. *Behavioural Brain Research*, *37*, 93-100.

Webster, W.G. (1990b). Concurrent cognitive processing and letter sequence transcription deficits in stutterers. *Canadian Journal of Psychology*, *44*(1), 1-13.

Webster, W.G. (1990c). Motor performance of stutterers: A search for mechanisms. *Journal of Motor Behavior, 22*, 553-571.

Webster, W.G. (1993). Hurried hands and tangled tongues: Implications of current research for the management of stuttering. In E. Boberg (Ed.), *The neuropsychology of stuttering* (pp. 73-127). Edmonton: University of Alberta Press.

Webster, W.G. (1997). Principles of human brain organization related to lateralization of language and speech motor functions in normal speakers and stutterers. In W. Hulstijn, H.F.M. Peters, & P.H.H.M. van Lieshout (Eds.), *Speech production: Motor control, brain research and fluency disorders* (pp. 119-139). Amsterdam: Elsevier.

Webster, W.G. (2004). From hand to mouth: Contributions of theory to evidenced-based treatment. In A. Bothe (Ed.), *Evidenced-Based Practice in Stuttering* (pp. 17-26). New York: Lawrence Erlbaum Associates.

Webster, W.G. (2013). Cultivating grass roots IPE: The Dalhousie University experience. *Journal of Interprofessional Care, 27*, 96-97.

Webster, W.G. & Poulos, M. (1987). Handedness distributions among adults who stutter. *Cortex, 23*, 705-708.

Webster, W.G. & Poulos, M. (1989). *Facilitating fluency: Transfer strategies for adult stuttering treatment programs.* Tucson, AZ: Communication Skill Builders, Inc. (Translated into Chinese and republished by Psychological Publishing Company, Taiwan. Reformatted and reprinted by Institute for Stuttering Treatment and Research, University of Alberta, Edmonton).

Webster, W.G. & Shoup, K. (1975). The development of paw preference in the rat following perinatal unilateral cortical ablations. *Perceptual and Motor Skills, 40*, 211-214.

Webster, W.G. & Thurber, D. (1978). Problem-solving strategies and manifest brain asymmetry. *Cortex,* **14,** 474-484.

Whillier, A., Hommel, S., Neef, N.E., Wolff von Gudenberg, A., Paulus, W., & Sommer, M. (2018). Adults who stutter lack the specialised pre-speech facilitation found in non-stutterers. PLoS ONE 13 (10): E0202634. https://doi.org/10.1371/journal.pone.0202634

Wise, S.P. (1984). The nonprimary motor cortex and its role in the cerebral control of movement. In G.M. Edelman, W.E. Gall, & W.M. Cowan (Eds.), *Dynamic aspects of neocortical function* (pp. 525-555). New York: John Wiley and Sons.

Wohlert, A.B. (1993). Event-related brain potentials preceding speech and nonspeech movements of varying complexity. *Journal of Speech and Hearing Research, 36,* 879-905.

Wolff, P.H., Hurwitz, I., & Moss, H. (1977). Serial organization of motor skills in left- and right-handed adults. *Neuropsychologia, 15,* 539-546.

Wu, J.C., Maguire, G., Riley, G., Fallon, J., LaCasse, L., Chin, S., Klein, E. Tang, C., Cadwell, S., & Lottenberg, S. (1995). A positron emission tomography [18]deoxyglucose study of developmental stuttering. *Neuroreport, 6,* 501-505.

Young, A. W. & Ratcliff, G. (1984). Visuospacial abilities of the right hemisphere. In Young, A.W. (Ed.), *Functions of the right cerebral hemisphere* (pp. 1-33). Orlando: Academic Press.

Young, R.M. (1970). *Mind, brain and adaptation in the nineteenth century.* Oxford University Press.

Zaidel, E. (1983). A response to Gazzaniga: Language in the right hemisphere, an empirical perspective. *American Psychologist, 38,* 542-546.

Other (Non-Cited) Publications by the Author

Furtado, J.C.S. & Webster, W.G. (1991). Concurrent language and motor task performance in bilinguals: A test of the age of acquisition hypothesis. *Canadian Journal of Psychology, 45,* 448-461.

Hranchuk, K., & Webster, W.G. (1975). Interocular transfer of lateral mirror-image discriminations by split-chiasm cats: Evidence of species differences. *Journal of Comparative and Physiological Psychology, 88,* 368-372.

Vaughn, C. & Webster, W.G. (1989). Bimanual handedness in adults who stutter. *Perceptual and Motor Skills, 68,* 375-382.

Webster, W.G. (1976). Conceptualizations of brain function. In M. Marx & F.A. Goodson (Eds.), *Theories of Contemporary Psychology,* 2nd edition (pp. 458-468). New York: Macmillan. (Reprinted from *Physiological Psychology,* 1973, *1,* 346-350).

Webster, W.G. (1977). Brain asymmetry in the rat: A new look at old data. *Neuropsychologia, 15,* 821-823.

Webster, W.G. (1977). Hemispheric asymmetry in cats. In S.R. Harnad, R.W. Doty, L. Goldstein, J. Jaynes, & G. Krathamer (Eds.), *Lateralization in the Nervous System. (*pp. 471-480). New York: Academic Press.

Webster, W.G. (1981). Morphological asymmetries of the cat brain. *Brain, Behavior and Evolution, 18,* 72-79.

Webster, W.G. (1987). What hurried hands reveal about "tangled tongues:" A neuropsychological approach to understanding stuttering. *Human Communication Canada, 11*(3), 11-18.

Webster, W.G. (1988). The use of scattergrams for the representation and analysis of lateralized interference effects in neuropsychology. *Canadian Journal of Psychology, 42,* 437-449.

Webster, W.G. (1990). Quality assurance: A framework for Canadian universities. *Canadian Journal of Higher Education, 20*(1), 75-85.

Webster, W.G. (1998). Brain models and the clinical management of stuttering. *Journal of Speech-Language Pathology and Audiology, 22,* 220-230.

Webster, W.G. & Godden-Webster, A.L. (2010). Stuttering. In Jung, J. H. et al., (Eds.), *Genetic Syndromes in Communication Disorders, 2nd edition* (pp. 186-191). Boston: College-Hill Press.

Webster, W.G. & Ryan, C.R.L. (1991). Task complexity and manual reaction times in stutterers. *Journal of Speech and Hearing Research*, *34*, 708-714.

Webster, W.G. & Webster, I.H. (1975). Anatomical asymmetry between the cerebral hemispheres of the cat brain. *Physiology and Behavior*, *14*, 867-869.

APPENDIX TABLES

Table 2: Examples of More-Effective, Less-Effective and Ineffective Self-Talk in Difficult Social and Speaking situations (from Webster & Poulos, 1989).

Preparing for speaking situations that may evoke anxiety

Ineffective ST	Less-effective ST	More-effective ST
"I can't cope."	"There's so much to do."	"The more I speak in this kind of situation, the easier it'll be to speak in similar situations in the future."
"What if I stutter?"	"There are so many people to speak to."	
"I can't imagine myself speaking in that situation."	"I have to do it."	
"My skills have never worked in this situation. I'm just too tense."	"Speaking is always frightening for me, but I'll do it this time."	"This situation will be an opportunity to practice by fluency skills."
"I've never done well in these situations. I should expect to bomb again."	"This situation will be a test to see if my fluency skills really work."	"I know ways to deal with this. I can use my fluency skills, relaxation skills, and think positive thoughts."
"I won't remember anything."	"I think I can handle it."	"I'll organize clearly what I must do. That'll help me remember."
"This is going to be a disaster."	"I can't forget what I need to say."	"I've used fluency skills before in situations like this one and can do so again."
"Nothing is going to help."	"I won't worry anymore."	"Time for a few controlled breaths so I'm comfortable and at ease.
	"Usually, some slow breathing lessens the anxiety."	

Table 2 (continued)(b)

Coping when speech anxiety starts to build

Ineffective S-T	Less-effective S-T	More-effective S-T
"Here comes the tension again."	"My muscles are getting tense. I must relax."	"My muscles are partially relaxed. Time to relax even more."
"I'm breaking down as usual."	"I won't stutter."	"Time to exaggerate fluency skills and remain in control."
"Another disaster in the making."	"This is frightening, but I think I'll be all right."	"I **can** meet this challenge."
"I'm not going to remember anything when I get up there to speak."	"I can't handle it unless I take one step at a time."	"One step at a time. "I can handle the situation by exaggerating my gentle onsets."
"Fluency skills won't work here. Why even bother to use them?"	"Don't get distracted. Don't forget to use fluency skills."	"I'll just monitor my breathing and gentle onsets. They help me start speaking fluently."
"What's the use of trying to say anything when I block like this?"	"If I block, I won't be able to make my point."	"I'm in control. Take a slow full breath and feel the relaxation."
"I can't stop this nervous feeling."	"Don't get nervous. You are in control."	"This is where I should gear down and monitor my breathing and onsets. They help me start more easily."
"I know I'm going to block on the first line."	"I'll just think about fluency skills."	

Table 2 (continued)(c)

Coping when speech anxiety starts to overwhelm

Ineffective S-T	Less-effective S-T	More-effective S-T
"I'm still nervous.	"Don't get nervous. You'll blow it."	"Right now, I feel nervous, but I can make myself feel calm and confident."
"It's not getting better."	"I really do hate having to speak."	
"Nothing is going to help my speech."	"I can beat this."	"The more I speak in this kind of situation, the easier it will be to speak the next time."
"I just want to get this over with."	"I shouldn't be afraid."	"I'll just pause and get myself organized. I can handle it."
"I have every right to hate speaking."	"I shouldn't let me anxiety show."	
"Everyone can see how anxious I feel."	"I've got to stop being afraid."	"I won't try to eliminate fear totally. I'll just keep it manageable."
"Nothing will help me stop this anxiety."	"Don't get angry."	"I'll pay attention to the present and what I have to say rather than imagining things that might happen."
"I've done it again!"	"The fluency skills don't work well when you really need them most."	
"Nothing will help."		"There's no point in getting angry. It won't help. Instead, I'll focus on being deliberate."

Table 2 (continued)(d)

Coping when it's all over and the anxiety has passed

Ineffective S-T	Less-effective S-T	More-effective S-T
"What a disaster. Thank goodness it's over! I'll never do that again."	"My speech wasn't perfect, and I had some disfluencies. I should have done better."	"My speech wasn't perfect, and I had some disfluencies, but that's okay. I tried, and that's what really counts."
"The audience must really have thought I was dumb when I blocked on that **D** sound."	"I wasn't a total success. Maybe next time I'll be better."	"I've succeeded in some ways, and I'll have these successes to draw on next time."
"People sure react when I use my fluency skills. Perhaps I shouldn't use them."	"Jim may have found my speech a little slow. I should have been more concerned about his reactions."	"I did the right things for myself. Jim may have found my speech a little slow but that's okay; I was comfortable."
"I hope there won't be a next time."	"I didn't think I would make it. I hope it's easier next time."	"That wasn't as hard as I thought. Next time it'll be easier."
"That was terrible."	"I'm not doing as well as I should."	"I'm doing better at this. I'm making progress."
"Never again, I hope."	"Thank goodness that's over."	"That was a good challenge and an opportunity to practice fluency skills."

Table 3: Self-Talk Analysis of Three Problem Situations
(from Webster and Poulos, 1989).

1. A situation involving time pressure

Tom had been using his fluency skills quite consistently during his day off and was quite pleased with his level of fluency. He decided to make a quick phone call to the store where he worked to check on his schedule. The person who answered the phone seemed rush; Tom imagined a hectic scene at the other end of the phone. He knew he should have been using fluency skills deliberately in the situation, but there were few if any fluency skills in his speech.

Here are some thoughts that might have led to Tom's reluctance or inability to use his fluency skills, and some more-effective alternatives.

Interfering thoughts	More-effective self-talk
"If I don't speak quickly, she'll think something is wrong with me."	"It doesn't matter what she thinks or how rushed she seems. I will continue to use my controlled breath and gentle onset skills because that's the most efficient way for me to communicate."
"I don't want her to be irritated with me so I'd better speak without fluency skills."	
"I don't think she likes it when I use my controlled speech techniques. I'd better speak spontaneously."	"Being fluent using fluency skills is more important than pleasing her. I really don't know how she feels about my speech. The important thing is that I get on with using my fluency skills."
"This person is in a terrible hurry and hasn't got time for my slow rate of speech with deliberate fluency skills."	"I won't imagine what is going on in the store. I'll concentrate on my speech and fluency skill use."
"I'll just get this over with quickly and be off to lunch."	"This is just a short call. Take your time and use fluency skills."

Table 3 (continued) (b)

"She expects quick answers, and if I use my controlled speech I won't appear as competent and sharp as she is."	"If she expects quick answers, that's her problem. I know what I'm doing. I can get my message across best by using my own style of speech."
"This situation is too rush, my heart is pounding, and I can't seem to be fluency skills started."	"The situation is rushed only when I make it that may. I need time to get started properly, so I'll concentrate on taking slow and controlled beaths and exaggerating my onsets."

* * * * * * *

2. A situation involving word avoidance

Cindy had been planning her first public speaking presentation. She had been having some difficulty achieving her fluency skills on some **S** and **F** sounds but decided to include words beginning with these sounds in her talk. On the day of her presentation, Cindy found that she used some of these words but consciously avoided others. She recognized that her first public speaking venture was a success, but she wanted to help herself eliminate the tendency to substitute words in future public speaking situation. She no longer wants to hold back.

Here are some thoughts that might have led to Cindy's reluctance or inability to use her fluency skills, and some more-effective alternatives.

Interfering thoughts	More-effective self-talk
"Despite my fluency course, I may stutter on some **S** or **F** sounds and that would ruin the presentation."	"Think back. I can make these sounds if I prepare for them by gearing down and using my fluency skills deliberately."

Table 3 (continued)(c)

"The audience will feel uncomfortable if I block. It'll be easier for everybody if I simply substitute some words."

"Even with deliberate fluency skills I can't make this sound all the time. I'd better use only sounds that I can make reliably."

"It's important to appear fluent if I'm so receive any respect."

"I'm going to block. Here comes an **S**-word again!"

"If I have problems with **S** and **F** sounds, people will laugh at me in their minds."

"I'll never be able to get **S** and **F** words easily."

"If I practice these sounds this time, it will be easier next time."

"I'd be pleased to have the audience know I can control my speech. I'd never have been able to stand up here six months ago."

"It's important for me to use fluency skills all the time, regardless of what others may think."

"In order to improve my fluency skills on **S** and **F** sounds, I need to practice saying words beginning with them, not avoid them, and this is a great opportunity practice them."

"I may have had some problem on that **S**-word, but at least I didn't avoid."

"I have some interesting information to give my audience, and they wouldn't be here if they didn't think it was interesting. The important thing is that I present my material the most effective way I can using my fluency skills. If it is less than perfect, it really doesn't matter."

* * * * * * * * *

Table 3 (continued)(d)

3. Meeting friends and family

After completing the intensive course, Carlos had been using fluency skills quite consistently both at home and at work. He found that being open about his speech techniques really helped him use them well. Carlos thought he had no reservations about using fluency skill but was surprised that he did not use speech fluency skills when bumped into an old friend downtown It happened again a week later when he visited his parents. His speech was completely spontaneous, even though he knew he should be using fluency skills which would control his speech. Carlos was upset and confused by his inconsistent use of fluency skills.

Here are some interfering thoughts that might have led to Carlos's reluctance or inability to use his fluency skills, and some more effective alternatives.

Interfering thoughts	More-effective self-talk
"I'm already comfortable with my friends and family. I don't need to use these fluency skills to be fluent."	"I've explained what I'm doing, and my family understands and supports me enthusiastically."
"I'll seem strange to my family and these old friends if I use controlled speech. I won't feel as comfortable and spontaneous as I would like to."	"I must resist spontaneous fluency. Controlled fluency is the only way to practice my fluency skills and firmly establish them in my speech."
"These old friends may think that my personality has changed along with my speech style, and I don't know what they may think of me."	"If these are my real friends, they won't be put off with my fluency skills and will know how much speaking fluently means to me."
"My parents and friends expected perfection, and I'd better be able to deliver it."	"Use fluency skills consistently and they will become natural."

www.ingramcontent.com/pod-product-compliance
Lightning Source LLC
Chambersburg PA
CBHW020316290526
45785CB00007B/2812